THE DOCTORS BOOK
OF
Home Remedies®
FOR
DEPRESSION

More Than 100 Solutions for Turning Your Life Around through Positive Thinking, Nutritional Healing, and More

By the Editors of *PREVENTION*.
Edited by Mary S. Kittel

RODALE

Cover Design: Lynn N. Gano and Tara Long

Library of Congress Cataloging-in-Publication Data

The doctors book of home remedies for depression : more than 100 solutions for turning your life around through positive thinking, nutritional healing, and more / by the editors of Prevention ; edited by Mary S. Kittel.

    p.   cm.
"Prevention Health Books"—T.p. verso.
Includes index.
ISBN 1–57954–232–8 paperback
    1. Depression, Mental—Popular works.   2. Depression, Mental—Alternative treatment. I. Kittel, Mary S.
II. Prevention Health Books. III. Prevention. IV. Title.
RC537 .D635   2001
616.85'2706—dc21   00–010496

Distributed to the book trade by St. Martin's Press

2   4   6   8   10   9   7   5   3   1   paperback

Visit us on the Web at www.rodaleremedies.com, or call us toll-free at (800) 848-4735.

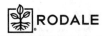

WE **INSPIRE** AND **ENABLE** PEOPLE TO IMPROVE
THEIR LIVES AND THE WORLD AROUND THEM

About *Prevention* Health Books

The editors of *Prevention* Health Books are dedicated to providing you with authoritative, trustworthy, and innovative advice for a healthy, active lifestyle. In all of our books, our goal is to keep you thoroughly informed about the latest breakthroughs in natural healing, medical research, alternative health, herbs, nutrition, fitness, and weight loss. We cut through the confusion of today's conflicting health reports to deliver clear, concise, and definitive health information that you can trust. And we explain in practical terms what each new breakthrough means to you, so you can take immediate, practical steps to improve your health and well-being.

Every recommendation in *Prevention* Health Books is based upon reliable sources, including interviews with qualified health authorities. In addition, we retain top-level health practitioners who serve on the Rodale Books Board of Advisors to ensure that all of the health information is safe, practical, and up-to-date. *Prevention* Health Books are thoroughly fact-checked for accuracy, and we make every effort to verify recommendations, dosages, and cautions.

The advice in this book will help keep you well-informed about your personal choices in health care—to help you lead a happier, healthier, and longer life.

Notice

This book is intended as a reference volume only, not as a medical manual. The information given here is designed to help you make informed decisions about your health. It is not intended as a substitute for any treatment that may have been prescribed by your doctor. If you suspect that you have a medical problem, we urge you to follow through with competent medical help.

The prescriptions in this book have specific instructions. Unless you are advised by a qualified practitioner, do not take higher dosages, mix the remedies with medications, or use the recommended herbs, essential oils, or supplements during pregnancy or while nursing. Always check with your doctor before beginning a new exercise program or if you experience any unfavorable reaction to a home remedy.

Permissions

Acknowledgments

Writers: Karen Cicero, Linda Formichelli, Brian Good, Kara M. Messinger, Judy West
Contributing Editor: Doug Dollemore
Editorial Researchers: Jan McLeod, Joanne D. Policelli

We would like to thank the following professionals for their health care advice: Jonathan Alpert, M.D., Ph.D.; Diane Austin; Paul Bergner; Harold Bloomfield, M.D.; Denise Borrelli; Roderick Borrie, Ph.D; Carol Boulware, Ph.D.; Richard Brown, M.D.; Hyla Cass, M.D.; Deepak Chopra, M.D.; Larry Christensen, Ph.D.; William G. Crook, M.D.; Carrie Demers, M.D.; Alice D. Domar, Ph.D.; Michele Wheat Dugan; James Duke, Ph.D.; Wayne W. Dyer, Ph.D.; Marcia Emery, Ph.D.; Paul J. Fitzgerald, Ph.D.; Ken Frey; Greg Garcia, N.D.; Joel Gavriele-Gold, Ph.D.; Geoffrey C. Godbey, Ph.D.; Jean Golding, Ph.D.; Karl Goodkin, M.D., Ph.D.; Kathleen Gould; Helen Graham; Bonnie M. Hagerty, Ph.D.; Judith Hall, Ph.D.; Richard Harte, PhD; Louise Hay; Christopher Hobbs; Michael J. Hurd, Ph.D; Margaret Jensvold, M.D.; Robert Kraut, Ph.D.; Daniel F. Kripke, M.D.; Denise Landau, Ph.D.; Deforia Lane, Ph.D; Derrick Lonsdale, M.D.; David Lykken, Ph.D.; John McIntyre, M.D.; Roger Mannell, Ph.D.; Lauren Marangell, M.D.; John Morreall, Ph.D; John Myerson, Ph.D.; David C. Nieman Dr.P.H.; Susan Nolan-Hoeksema, Ph.D.; Patricia Norris, Ph.D.; Michele E. Novotni, Ph.D.; Robert Oresick, Ph.D.; James Penland, Ph.D.; Joseph Pizzorno, N.D.; Gerrold Rosenbaum, M.D.; Dannel I. Schwartz; Daniel L. Segal, Ph.D.; Norman Shealy, M.D., Ph.D.; Mark Sisti, Ph.D.; Elizabeth Somer, R.D.; Malcolm Southwood; Andrew Stoll, M.D.; Fred Straussburger, Ph.D.; Maryann Troiani; Andrew Weil, M.D.; Melvyn R. Werbach, M.D; Redford Williams, M.D.; Reg A. Williams, Ph.D.; Judith Wurtman, Ph.D.; Janet Zand, O.M.D.

Contents

CHANGE YOUR MOOD BY CHANGING YOUR MIND 71

Cognitive therapists challenge you to examine and exorcise your negative thinking patterns. Free yourself from distorted ideas, clobber self-defeating thoughts, and pump up your self-esteem. Gain the peace of mind you've wanted all your life by finally accepting your limitations—as well as your well-deserved lovability.

RELAX AND ENJOY LIFE 91

Insist on being surrounded by the people, environment, and activities that make you vibrant, while avoiding habits and traps that bring you down. And if you occasionally do slip into the frazzled zone, learn to create your own personal spa with the experts' master mood-soothing remedies.

ALTERNATIVE OPTIONS 119

When you need to talk to someone with a fresh perspective or are seeking someone to gently ease the hurt, consider the holistic healers in this miniguide. Music therapists, acupuncturists, intuitive healers, and other alternative health practitioners are uniquely trained to help bring relief for your headaches and heartaches.

INDEX 129

Braving
the Storm

Have we lost our heads, writing a home remedies book for depression? Although experts consider depression the "common cold" of mental health, we realize that this topic is far more challenging than the sniffles and aches for which our famous home remedy gurus give quick and natural solutions.

Depression affects nearly 10 percent of adult Americans, and major depression is the leading cause of disability in the United States and worldwide. It can be wrenching to your relationships; disrupt your eating and sleeping habits; impair your reasoning, memory, concentration, and sexual ability; and increase your risk for heart disease, accidents, substance abuse, and death. Without proper treatment, painful symptoms can endure for months, years, or a lifetime.

Actually, the frequency and severity of the problem is all the more reason that we wanted to write a home remedies book on depression—when you have it, you need to take better care of yourself than ever. What could be more appropriate than a book that will help you clear up what's stressful in your lifestyle, power up your diet, and offer positive ways to resolve problems?

Whether you are struggling your way out of the grief of a recent loss, have seasonal or occasional bouts of the blues, or have a clinically diagnosed depressive illness, we believe that you will find it refreshing to know how you can take a proactive approach, using hundreds of proven and practical methods.

What's more, you can and will feel better. Experts will

tell you that *once properly diagnosed*, even the most severe forms of depression are highly manageable and very treatable.

The first steps are to determine if you need a doctor's help and find out how to get a diagnosis. If you are diagnosed with depressive illness, you will find that many of the 100-plus techniques in this book can ingeniously enhance the treatment prescribed by your doctor. If your blues are temporary or mild, this book is loaded with nondrug strategies to facilitate a speedy and full recovery.

Know the Signs

Depression can come on suddenly, seemingly for no reason or as the result of a stressful or life-altering event. It can also grow slowly over months and years, gradually draining away happiness and hope.

"The illness creates the same kinds of painful feelings that you'd experience after a death in the family, a failed romance, a lost job, a serious illness, or any other life crisis that leaves you feeling sad, lonely, or 'down' for a period of time," explains Jonathan Alpert, M.D., Ph.D., assistant professor of psychology at Harvard Medical School and associate director of the Depression Clinical and Research Program at Massachusetts General Hospital in Boston. "The difference is that while you generally recover from most stressful events like a death or other serious loss within a period of months, depression often refuses to go away on its own." Instead it persists, getting in the way of your job or relationships with family and friends, and basically prevents you from getting on with your life.

Although it can take many forms, here are some common symptoms of depression.

- Persistent sadness
- Loss of self-confidence

- Feelings of hopelessness or helplessness
- Numbness (lack of feelings or emotions)
- Lethargy or increased lack of energy or drive
- Insomnia or problems getting up in the morning
- Persistent headaches, stomachaches, backaches, or muscle or joint pain
- Increased difficulty making decisions
- Problems remembering things or concentrating
- Loss of interest in pleasurable activities, including hobbies, sports, and sex
- Increased isolation from friends and family members
- Eating disturbances (weight gain or weight loss)
- Panic attacks
- Overwhelming feelings of guilt or fear
- Frequent crying
- Increased arguments with friends or coworkers
- Loss of interest in saving money or controlling how much you spend
- Dangerous or compulsive risk taking
- Thoughts of your own death or suicide

To be clinically diagnosed as having depression, you have to have a depressed mood or loss of interest in ordinary activities for at least 2 weeks, plus four or more of the symptoms of depression listed above. If you fit this description, see your primary care doctor as soon as possible.

Before making an official diagnosis, your doctor will want to rule out any illness that may cause similar symptoms, such as thyroid conditions, lupus, multiple sclerosis, or diabetes. Hidden Mood Benders on page 11 will help you identify other possible underlying causes of your discontent.

Depression may be missed because its complex and varied symptoms often confuse family doctors who aren't in the practice of looking for it. So, if you suspect depression, ask your family doctor to do a specific evaluation for it.

If you can't get the help that you may feel you need, search your telephone directory under "mental health," "social services," "crisis prevention," or "hotlines" for a psychiatrist, psychologist, or counselor who can give you immediate attention. Hospital emergency rooms can also provide temporary help for an emotional problem, and their staff can tell you how and where to get further help.

It's Not in Your Head

Whatever you do, don't avoid treatment because of someone else's ignorance. The fact is, we live in a culture that harbors unfair misconceptions, such as the belief that depression is a sign of weakness or that the depressed person should "just snap out of it." Nothing could be further from the truth.

The first idea to hold on to is that it's not your fault.

For starters, the hormonal system that regulates the body's responses to stress is often persistently overactive in many patients with depression, which may explain classic symptoms like edginess, moodiness, or sexual impairment. The mood-altering hormonal fluctuations of the menstrual cycle, pregnancy, childbirth, menopause, and oral contraceptives help explain why women experience depression almost twice as often as men do. Shifts in hormone levels also are also a suspected factor in depression being a common problem for teenagers, since major depression typically begins between the ages of 15 and 30.

Modern brain-imaging technology offers a visual picture of how the neural circuits responsible for moods, thinking, sleep, appetite, and behavior may not function properly in depressed people, or it may show that chemical messengers called neurotransmitters are impaired.

Although there are more than 80 different types of neurotransmitters in the human brain, a select few of these chemicals seem to have more control than others over mental functioning. They include epinephrine, histamine, dopamine, endorphins, and serotonin, which work together in a delicate balance to help you concentrate, remember, and perform other mental tasks. Many of the most popular antidepressant drugs are targeted to regulate those neurotransmitters.

As far as how biological irregularities develop in the first place, experts believe that both genetics and certain lifestyle factors make people more vulnerable. "Some people are genetically predisposed through family history to be depressed," says Fred Straussburger, Ph.D., a clinical psychologist based in McLean, Virginia. "It can be the result of an abnormality in the family's biology that might make them more susceptible to the disease, or it could be something environmental about the way your family operates or conditions in which children were raised." If you come from a family with a history of mental illness, you are about two times more likely than someone else to suffer from depression.

The environmental factors suspected of breeding depression include how much day-to-day conflict we experience and how we react to it. Stress is one of the primary causes of depression in the United States, says Susan Nolan-Hoeksema, Ph.D., professor of psychology at the University of Michigan in Ann Arbor.

Major depression is more common in cities than in rural areas, partly due to the increased agitation of dealing with traffic, crime, and high-pressure lifestyles. "Most people with depression don't have to look very far into their personal lives to find that they feel overwhelmed by events and situations that they think are controlling them," says Dr. Nolan-Hoeksema.

Social isolation is another liability. This is illustrated in the high incidence of depression among elderly people who are "shut in" and teens who consider themselves unable to "fit in."

Hope lies in the promise that the more we understand the factors that contribute to an emotional disorder, the more control we can have over reducing or preventing our vulnerability to depression. For example, research shows that people who exercise regularly over a long period of time have far fewer bouts of depression than people who exercise infrequently or not at all. It is highly likely that this physical release is beneficial because it lessens some of the stress factors mentioned above.

Treatment and Self-Help

Traditional treatment for clinical depression combines talk therapy, peer support groups, and prescriptions for antidepressant drugs like fluoxetine (Prozac), sertraline (Zoloft), and paroxetine (Paxil), although medication is increasingly becoming the primary if not the sole thrust of mainstream treatment.

The most popular medications are designed to compensate for the imbalance of neurotransmitters in the brain. Since different drugs are suitable for different people, it is not uncommon to test six or more medications in the first year of treatment. Each drug may take 8 weeks to produce any therapeutic benefit. As with all treatment options, you can expect your mood to improve gradually, not immediately. Feeling better takes time, so experts strongly encourage you to stay on your medication and not stop taking prescribed drugs on your own.

A nondrug approach. Herbs can support you in battling depression by increasing energy, bringing calm, and working similarly to antidepressant drugs by regulating neurotransmitters. Natural supplements like SAM-e, 5-HTP, and St. John's wort are gaining popularity for providing a gentle mood lift, but unlike antidepressants, they have few side effects such as drowsiness, nausea, or sexual impairment. In Germany, prescriptions are written for St. John's wort 20 times more frequently than for Prozac.

Nowadays, you can pick up a bottle of supplements just about anywhere, from the supermarket to the spa, but doctors urge you not to experiment without their blessing.

"Certain supplements may interact with the medications your doctor has prescribed, or, if you avoid seeing a physician, you may not find out if your depression symptoms have another cause, such as thyroid disease," points out Lauren Marangell, M.D., director of the center for mood disorders at Baylor College of Medicine in Houston.

If you're having trouble locating a doctor who is knowledgeable about both pharmaceutical medications and natural supplements, contact the American Holistic Medical Association at 6728 Old McLean Village Drive, McLean, VA 22101, or log on to its Web site at www.holisticmedicine.org.

Nutritional therapy. A healthy diet is vital for more than keeping up your immunity and energy during times of stress. With depression, as with any other illness, you can count on food (and nutritional supplements) to support healing. Fresh greens and sunflower seeds, for example, are rich in compounds like tryptophan, lithium, omega-3 fatty acids, and phenylalanine—compounds that have a direct impact on mood. Solid evidence shows that taking nutrients such as vitamins B_6, B_{12}, and C as well as zinc, magnesium, thiamin, and folic acid has relieved depression. In fact, some doctors prescribe vitamins and minerals for their psychiatric patients to enhance the effects of pharmaceutical treatments. See Diet, Herbs, and Supplements on page 33 for guidance in making wise food and nutrition choices for your specific needs.

Emotional disclosure. According to research at Duke University in Durham, North Carolina, talking with friends, confiding in a therapist, praying, and writing about your thoughts are all highly beneficial physically and mentally.

"There are several reasons why emotional disclosure is so effective," explains Daniel L. Segal, Ph.D., assistant professor of psychology at the University of Colorado at Colorado Springs. "When you have something distressing on your mind and you try to not think about it, that takes physiological work and causes stress on your body." If you can let out those thoughts in a structured way, you can reduce stress on your body and often put the distressing thoughts in a context where it's easier to see solutions, he says.

You will find many writing exercises throughout this book, along with specific steps to open the lines of communication with loved ones and strangers and even how to rediscover your spiritual side.

Cognitive therapy. Cognitive therapies help a person to change the negative styles of thinking and behaving that are associated with depression. Researchers at the University of British Columbia in Vancouver analyzed 28 separate studies to determine how people fared after different types of mental health therapy. Those who used cognitive therapy did better than 98 percent of those who had no other therapy, better than 70 percent of those who took antidepressant drugs, and better than 70 percent of those who tried traditional talk therapy.

You don't necessarily need to pay a cognitive therapist to get results. Support groups will probably catch your negative thinking patterns, and Change Your Mood by Changing Your Mind on page 71 provides exercises to examine and empower your attitude.

Get physical. Nothing is more widely agreed upon among health care practitioners than the value of regular exercise for emotional health. Whether you consult a psychologist, a family physician, or an alternative health practitioner, you will likely find a workout program high on your treatment list. We could go into elaborate explanations of how exercise releases feel-good chemicals or improves blood circulation to the brain, but you already know the most common and most valuable denominator—it makes you feel good. Walking is a favored activity among the experts interviewed for this book, but all agree that the sport or activity should be whatever appeals to you the most. See Relax and Enjoy Life on page 91 to motivate you to start moving, and for other tips for a good-mood lifestyle.

Self-nurturing. Alternative health techniques like music therapy and aromatherapy are not only safe and easy, they are also fun to experiment with. Better yet, science is beginning to recognize the value of these more "touchy-feely" approaches to well-being.

In a Japanese study, 12 depressed men who were treated with citrus fragrance (aromatherapy) for 11 weeks were able to dramatically decrease their doses of antidepressants. Researchers say that massage can release beneficial chemicals like serotonin, which antidepressants work to enhance, and reduce levels of norepinephrine and cortisol, which anxiety medications attempt to lower. Treat yourself to some of the suggestions for relaxation and nurturing in Relax and Enjoy Life, or check Alternative Options on page 119 to find a holistic health practitioner who aims to soothe your psyche in the spirit of love and hope.

"When diagnosed accurately and treated with either antidepressant medication or one of the many nondrug therapies, there is virtually no one who cannot be helped," says John McIntyre, M.D., past president of the American Psychiatric Association. "Feel free to try as many things as you can, because while depression can be a debilitating illness, if it is properly treated, your chances of making a complete recovery from the condition are very good."

Hidden Mood Benders

"*Although the world is full of suffering, the world is full of overcoming it.*"

—Helen Keller, *American author and inspirational speaker admired for her courage, faith, and determination to transcend the physical challenges of blindness and deafness.*

EXIT THE ZOMBIE ZONE

Just because the rest of the world seems to be running on empty doesn't mean that it's healthy for you to miss your 8 hours of sleep.

America is the land of the sleep deprived. Nowhere else in the world is it fashionable to brag about getting just a few hours of sleep a night. Even if it's become somewhat of a cultural norm, catching just 4 or 5 hours of sleep is reckless, and, for some, the constant physical depletion can lead to or aggravate depression.

"Your body needs 8 to 10 hours of sleep, and it needs that sleep each and every night," says Denise Landau, Ph.D. "If you're not getting that amount of sleep, you're not going to be functioning fully at work or in your personal life, and, ultimately, the quality of life is going to suffer."

If you always feel drained or you tend to fall asleep in awkward places like a quiet waiting room, in church, or on a plane, you're probably sleep deprived. And although it sounds pretty obvious, the key to fighting the problem is just training yourself to go to bed on time.

"Lay down the law to get yourself under the covers at a regular hour each night; your body will take care of everything else," says Dr. Landau.

—Denise Landau, Ph.D., *is a clinical psychologist in Memphis.*

SNORING IS NOTHING TO SNEEZE AT

An untreated case of sleep apnea may be the major cause of depression in your life.

Sleep apnea, a condition that causes people to stop breathing for several seconds at a time while asleep, not only leads to fatigue and a general lack of energy but can also be an often-undiagnosed cause of some forms of mild depression.

"When a person undergoes an episode of sleep apnea, the brain is deprived of oxygen for a short period of time," explains Daniel F. Kripke, M.D. "It's this lack of oxygen that causes symptoms of depression."

Sleep apnea–induced depression may show up as a tendency to wake during the night, changes in appetite, loss of interest in sex, and a generally negative outlook on life.

Ask your sleeping partner to listen to you or tape record you while you are asleep. Any loud snoring or unusual breathing sounds should make you suspect sleep apnea. If you're overweight or just don't feel well-rested even after a full night's sleep, it's a good idea to test yourself, explains Dr. Kripke.

If you think that you may have apnea, it's best to see a doctor, although losing weight and using anti-snoring products can help you fend off symptoms.

—Daniel F. Kripke, M.D., *is professor of psychiatry at the University of California, San Diego, School of Medicine.*

DON'T DIET YOUR WAY TO DEPRESSION

Worries over how much or how little you should be eating can become a major source of depression.

As a rule, almost all people with eating disorders of any kind end up depressed at some point. Whether you overeat or undereat, you may endure uncomfortable feelings of obsession over body image and desperation about trying to change the reading on your scale. Anything that creates such stress in your life can become a source of depression, says Jonathan Alpert, M.D., Ph.D.

In addition, severe or yo-yo dieting can cause nutritional deficiencies, dehydration, and chemical imbalances that can contribute to mental illness. Worse yet, full-fledged eating disorders can lead to such serious damage to your vital organs that you are at risk for stroke and even death.

"Usually, it's a guess as to whether it's an eating disorder that's causing depression or whether it's depression that's causing the eating disorder. It can go either way," says Dr. Alpert.

If you suspect that you are developing an eating disorder, it is imperative that you seek advice from a counselor. Also consider looking in your local newspaper for meetings of Overeaters Anonymous or check the Web site of the American Anorexia Bulimia Association at www.aabainc.org for more information.

—Jonathan Alpert, M.D., Ph.D., *is assistant professor of psychology at Harvard Medical School and associate director of the Depression Clinical and Research Program at Massachusetts General Hospital in Boston.*

AVOID A PRESCRIPTION FOR THE BLUES

The medications you take to stay healthy might be limiting your health in other ways.

Depression is a fairly common side effect of many drugs, including everything from caffeine and alcohol to prescription medications like sleeping pills, birth control pills, and inhalants. It's also especially common with many blood pressure medications, says Robert Oresick, Ph.D.

Fortunately, Dr. Oresick says, tracing the source of the problem is generally a straightforward procedure. The symptoms associated with medication-induced depression would be typical of other forms of depression, including low energy levels, fatigue, loss of sex drive, and decreased interest in formerly enjoyable activities.

"All you really have to do is look at the medication you're taking and the length of time you've been taking it, then compare that information with the amount of time since you last remember feeling really good," says Dr. Oresick. "If, on the other hand, you've been taking a drug for years and your depressive symptoms started a few months ago, you need to look for other potential sources of depression."

If you believe that a medication may be to blame for your depression, Dr. Oresick says it's time to talk to your doctor about adjusting your dosage or possibly even changing your prescription to a different drug.

—Robert Oresick, Ph.D., *is associate dean in the department of psychology at Boston University.*

CLEAR THE AIR

Something as seemingly innocent as aerosols or air fresheners may be polluting your spirits.

The next time you find yourself reaching for that can of air freshener, keep this in mind: Your efforts to make your home or office smell a little better may be having a negative impact on your health.

In a survey of 14,000 women in the United Kingdom, researchers found that being exposed to air fresheners or aerosols on a daily basis increased levels of depression by almost 20 percent and increased the number of headaches the women experienced by more than 25 percent.

"Aerosols and air fresheners contain dozens of volatile organic compounds like zylene, ketones, and aldehydes, all of which can be toxic in high doses," says Jean Golding, Ph.D., author of the study. Dr. Golding speculates that these compounds weaken the body's defenses, making people easier targets for depression.

"We need to research the phenomenon further, but until then, I wouldn't use aerosols or air fresheners, especially if I were trying to battle the effects of depression," she says.

As alternatives to commercial sprays, natural essential oils can refresh the air, and aromatherapists say that scents such as rose geranium, citrus, and jasmine will also boost your mood. You can purchase the natural oils at health food stores along with a diffuser, aroma lamp, or perfume lantern to heat them.

—Jean Golding, Ph.D., *is an epidemiologist at the University of Bristol in England.*

CHECK YOUR THYROID

A malfunctioning gland could be mistaken for clinical depression.

Are you experiencing mental sluggishness, little or no libido, irritability, poor eating and sleeping habits, memory loss, or feelings of weakness and fatigue most of the time? While it's true that these are symptoms of clinical depression, they are also signs of a malfunctioning thyroid gland.

Your thyroid is located just under the skin of your neck, below your Adam's apple. When it's in top form, it regulates growth, maturation, and the speed of your metabolism through the release of certain hormones. A thyroid malfunction, however, can lead to a host of problems, including some that sound uncannily like depression.

An underactive thyroid causes a condition called hypothyroidism, which may cause swelling at the site of the gland at the base of your neck. But even before the gland enlarges, hypothyroidism often shows up in symptoms such as unexplained weight gain and fatigue. You may experience other physical symptoms that include thinning hair, dry skin, a puffy face, slowed speech, and feeling cold all the time, in addition to the psychological signs mentioned above, says Andrew Weil, M.D.

Hyperthyroidism, a condition in which the thyroid is overactive, can lead to mood swings, anxiety, and other depressive traits. You may also experience sudden weight loss, moist skin and increased sweating, shakiness, or sensitivity to bright light and heat.

"If you have symptoms of either condition, you should talk to your doctor about being tested," says Dr. Weil. There are medications or supplements that bring an underactive thyroid back to normal (see "Keep Your Eye on Iodine" on page 58), and surgery can correct an overactive gland.

—Andrew Weil, M.D., *is director of the program in integrative medicine and clinical professor of medicine at the University of Arizona College of Medicine in Tucson and author of many books on holistic health, including* Eating Well for Optimum Health.

IS WINTER MAKING YOU SAD?

Lack of sunlight may make you feel like you want to crawl under a rock, and for good reason.

Seasonal affective disorder (SAD) is a form of depression triggered by the lack of full-intensity sunlight during the darker winter months. It can begin as early as August or September of each year and is believed to be related to the hibernation response in some animals. Just like a bear whose metabolism slows down for the winter, people who are affected by SAD begin to notice a general loss of energy, a lack of motivation, and an increased desire to sleep.

It's estimated that 25 million Americans get the "winter blues," and 10 million suffer from severe SAD. If you work odd shifts, spend a majority of your time indoors, or live in a far northern climate where there are more cloudy days than sunny ones, you're highly susceptible to this illness. Psychologists can formally diagnose SAD (one clinical marker is abnormal levels of the sleep-regulating hormone melatonin), but you can figure that you probably have it if you notice an annual recurrence of negative emotions and lethargy at a specific time of the year, says Andrew Weil, M.D. Another distinguishing trait is a constant craving for carbohydrates in the winter, which probably means that you tend to overeat at that time.

If you suspect that you have SAD, there are lots of techniques to help relieve the symptoms—everything from getting more outdoor exercise in peak sunlight hours to changing to full-spectrum lighting (see page 106 for instructions on using light therapy). Some doctors also recommend taking the herb St. John's wort. If you're still feeling down, they can prescribe antidepressants during the darker months of the year (see page 64 for more information on taking St. John's wort).

For more information on managing this disorder, contact the National Organization for SAD at P.O. Box 40133, Washington, DC 20016.

—Andrew Weil, M.D., *is director of the program in integrative medicine and clinical professor of medicine at the University of Arizona College of Medicine in Tucson and author of many books on holistic health, including* Eating Well for Optimum Health.

DETOX GENTLY

*Ending a depressive addiction can leave
you feeling . . . depressed?*

Addiction to alcohol or drugs is a sure precursor to depression, but what many people don't expect is that kicking a bad habit—whether it's a major addiction such as alcohol or prescription pills or a more common one such as caffeine or nicotine—can also lead to an emotional slump.

"For many people, withdrawal from any sort of chemical addiction triggers a depressive episode," says Gerrold Rosenbaum, M.D. "That depression can be caused by your body's physical craving for the drug you were addicted to or by the sense of loss or deprivation that you feel since you no longer have that drug to help you escape other problems in your life."

Either way, there is a lot you can do to help yourself through the process. To replace the chemical calm you were dependent on, engage in the exercise, meditation, and breathing techniques suggested in this book. And eating at least three to five daily servings of fruits and vegetables and drinking at least eight 8-ounce glasses of water daily will help move the addictive substance out of your body and rebuild your natural vitality.

—Gerrold Rosenbaum, M.D., *is professor of psychiatry at Harvard Medical School.*

ALLERGIC TO HAPPINESS?

*Your emotional slump could be a result
of a covert food reaction.*

A piece of warm bread or a couple of cookies may seem like a good way to make your bad feelings go away, but those "comfort" foods that you rely on to get you through tough times may be the very thing responsible for your depression.

"Research shows that many of the symptoms related to depression can be reactions to food," says William G. Crook, M.D., "yet this relationship between food and mood is often overlooked by physicians."

The reason for this, according to Dr. Crook, is that some food allergies and sensitivities cannot be detected by conventional allergy skin tests. Instead, they must be identified by a carefully followed elimination diet.

"In addition to low moods, if you suffer from persistent fatigue, muscle pain, memory loss, or chronic infections, or you have problems sleeping or concentrating at work, you may have a food allergy that's causing those symptoms," says Dr. Crook.

To identify the culprit, Dr. Crook suggests using the following strategy during a period of several weeks when you won't be traveling and that doesn't include major holidays.

• For 1 week, strictly avoid these suspect foods: soft drinks, wheat, chocolate, and sugar; anything made with milk or yeast; and any food containing food colorings or other additives, flavorings, or preservatives.

• Limit your diet to vegetables and fruit (except corn and citrus fruits); meats (except bacon, sausage, hot dogs, and lunchmeat); unprocessed grains (oats, brown rice, and barley); and water.

• When the week is over, consider your symptoms. If you have followed the diet strictly and the depression and other symptoms have lifted, it's likely that you have a food allergy. If you don't feel different, add common foods that you eat more than once a week to the suspect list and eliminate them for 1 week.

• Begin adding one suspect food a day back into your diet. Keep track of the foods and when you add them. If your symptoms return, you'll know which food you're sensitive to.

• Keep the offending food out of your diet or seek a holistic health practitioner's help in building your resistance to it, and you should return to normal health.

—William G. Crook, M.D., *is a physician in Jackson, Tennessee, and author of several natural health books, including* The Yeast Connection.

ACCEPT YOUR EMOTIONS

*Unfortunately, life provides a bounty
of distractions if you want to hide
from emotional pain. But rather than
being liberating, evasiveness can
be lethal.*

To some degree, we all have a tendency to make ourselves superbusy while waiting in vain for somebody to fix our problems or hoping that they'll go away on their own. Unfortunately, not only does internalizing negative emotions cause them to fester and build, but numerous medical studies now confirm that untended stress and anger can increase your risk for cancer, stroke, heart disease, and yes, clinical depression.

If you find yourself socializing, watching more television than usual, or even reading ferociously to "escape" your problems, you may be on a dangerous path. Giving up claim to painful feelings is actually giving up your power to heal from them.

"Remind yourself often that ultimately, you are the creator of your own reality. You are the interpreter, the seer, the decision-maker, and the chooser," says Deepak Chopra, M.D. Here are his techniques for facing the cause of your unhappiness and turning it around.

• Instead of telling yourself that an emotion is bad, ask what it has to tell you. Every emotion exists for a reason, and the reason can always help you spiritually grow.

• Instead of pushing an emotion away, take a closer look at it. Very often, you will find that emotions are layered. Anger masks fear; fear masks hurt. Facing your fears means getting through the layers to the root, where real healing can occur.

• If you find yourself starting to say, "I can't let go of my feelings," don't believe it. Resisting only makes things worse. Let the emotions rise. Release them by crying, screaming, losing your temper, shaking with fear—whatever it takes. Emotions come and go. Each one has a rhythm, so let yourself be in that rhythm. The best way not to drown is to ride the wave.

• If a feeling is overwhelming, say to yourself, "I want to ride this out a bit longer before I look at it." Realize that the overwhelming feeling isn't the real you; it's something you're going through (see "Air Out the Skeletons in Your Closet" on page 28 for help if a past traumatic event comes up).

• If you recognize that certain situations always bring the same reaction, ask what you need to learn in order for that reaction to change. Repetition is like a knock on the door—it stops when you open the door and greet what is on the other side.

    —Deepak Chopra, M.D., *is director for educational programs at The Chopra Center for Well Being in La Jolla, California. He has written many books on holistic health, including* Body, Mind, and Soul: The Seven Spiritual Laws of Success.

MANAGE YOUR GRIEF

Dealing with the death of a friend or family member shouldn't take over your life.

Bereavement is a tender and necessary passage that's part of being human. Experiencing a gripping sense of loss is healthy, as long as the intensity gradually wanes.

According to Paul J. Fitzgerald, Ph.D., it's the pain and feelings of loss that linger months after a death that are the most harmful to people, and those feelings often lead to mild to moderate forms of depression.

"Generally, the amount of time it takes to successfully come to terms with the death of someone close to you is 3 to 4 months," says Dr. Fitzgerald. "After that time, the pain shouldn't be so debilitating that you can't function. If it is, that's when it's time for you to seek some sort of counseling."

One of the best things you can do to deal with your emotions in a time of loss is to join a support group. "Friends and family members may be able to help as well, but since they may be facing the same loss, you're likely to have the best luck with outsiders who can impartially look at the situation and help you to come to terms with it."

—Paul J. Fitzgerald, Ph.D., *is a licensed clinical psychologist based in Lyons, Illinois.*

SICK OF THE SIDELINES?

*Lacking quality relationships and a
sense of belonging to a community is a
potential risk factor for depression.*

Having friends and a strong social support network is vital to our mental health. That much is well-demonstrated in a significant amount of research.

Bonnie M. Hagerty, Ph.D., lead author of one such study, stresses that it's not just the number of friends and family members you have or how busy your social life is that prevents and relieves depression. Now we understand better that what's really important is our sense of belonging and the extent to which we feel valued and needed by our family and friends.

Ask yourself a few questions, such as, "Whom do I trust with my feelings? Who would feel free to come to me in the middle of the night just to talk?" If you're not satisfied with the answers, you may need to create better connections.

At parties or other social situations, focus on making other people feel good about themselves. The next time you're out, introduce yourself to someone and consciously make an effort to keep the conversation focused on that person's interests. This is the way to develop habits that will help you feel better about yourself and make new friends.

Each day, try to talk to a person whom you rarely speak to. If you can't get out, you can rely on the telephone or the Internet to socialize.

—Bonnie M. Hagerty, Ph.D., *is associate professor at the School of Nursing of the University of Michigan in Ann Arbor.*

AIR OUT THE SKELETONS IN YOUR CLOSET

A traumatic childhood event, even a seemingly forgotten one, could keep you on an emotional downswing for decades.

Many people experience traumatic events early in their lives, such as abuse, divorce, deaths, and so on (big "T" traumas), or parental criticism, excessive control, neglect, and similar situations (small "t" traumas), says Carol Boulware, Ph.D.

Whatever the event was, it's possible that the negative feelings you experienced during that time became trapped in your unconscious memory system, lingering there for years and bringing about unidentifiable feelings of anxiety, depression, or low self-esteem.

"These unconscious negative memories are often reactivated later in life when similar situations occur," says Dr. Boulware. Once triggered, the old unconscious memory system generates the same amounts of fear, guilt, or anger that you felt at the time of the original event, and they can resurface as anxiety, depression, or low self-esteem. These old unconscious negative memories are the skeletons in your emotional closet!

When strong negative feelings occur, Dr. Boulware recommends the following steps.

• Try to recognize what immediate issue is triggering their release, such as issues of excessive responsibility, vulnerability, the need for control or a lack of control, or feelings of being defective.

• How old do you feel? Are you acting like a child? If so, the feelings are probably emotional skeletons.

• Tell yourself that you now have other choices.

• Behave the way that you think is appropriate, regardless of the feelings you are experiencing.

• Later, sit down and think about the origins of the emotional skeleton. Identify earlier life experiences that generated the same feelings.

• Once you've identified the source of the feelings, imagine yourself in that situation again. This time, though, envision yourself doing what you now know would have been appropriate, or bringing in an adult who could have stopped the situation from occurring.

• Journaling, imagining different outcomes, or talking with a friend about these past events is often very helpful in gradually removing the emotional skeleton from your closet.

According Dr. Boulware, just knowing that the emotional skeleton exists and what its origins are can do wonders for changing existing feelings and behaviors. "If, however, these tips are not enough, seek professional help, especially with someone who is experienced in working with past traumatic experiences," she says. "I have found EMDR therapy (Eye Movement Desensitization and Reprocessing therapy) to be especially helpful in removing emotional skeletons from my clients' closets."

—Carol Boulware, Ph.D., *is a clinical psychotherapist and EMDR Level II Trained Therapist in Los Angeles.*

BLAST AWAY CYNICISM

It's time to face up to the fact that your critical disposition doesn't make you very good company for yourself or anyone else.

"Cheer up. The worst is yet to come," advised a 1920s comic. Playful irony is healthy, but if you really do carry around callous hopelessness or your cynical remarks (even disguised as humor) really do reflect your hostility, you may be sending yourself on a downslide.

When you find the worst in people and situations, it creates a vacuum inside you that can only be filled with anger, impatience, anxiety, and loneliness. On the other hand, the more you practice not criticizing and not complaining, the more the vacuum within you will fill with love and appreciation, explains Wayne W. Dyer, Ph.D.

Since cynicism is a defense mechanism that prevents you from fostering new bonds with people, a key to breaking out of it is to cultivate the subtle human connections that are available to you every day. Deciding to overcome your grim approach to life will allow uplifting energy to come pouring into your life.

Dr. Dyer recommends the following shift in focus to help you develop a more fulfilling attitude.

• Recognize the reality that virtually everything that you possess is a result of the efforts of others. Your home, meals, clothing, entertainment, and transportation, the talents you have learned, and yes, even your body, are all, in some way, gifts from others.

Remind yourself every day that the efforts of thousands and thousands of people are working in harmony to fulfill both your basic needs and your pleasures, says Dr. Dyer.

• Give yourself a specific period of time, perhaps 30 days, to try avoiding complaining and fault finding. Catch yourself when you are about to find fault with someone or some situation and replace the negativity with a statement of compassion. For example, consider that a performer who's getting feedback from his microphone must be very embarrassed, rather than blurting out something like, "There are idiots running this show."

• To go a step further, don't underestimate the power of doing small acts of kindness. Favors like bringing your neighbor his newspaper or telling a waitress how much you appreciate her attention to details will warm up your life with positive feelings. You may find that you'll have no room in your life for cynicism.

—Wayne W. Dyer, Ph.D., *is a lecturer in the field of self-empowerment and author of many best-selling self-help classics, including* Manifest Your Destiny: The Nine Spiritual Principles of Getting Everything You Want.

GOT THE SPACE AGE BLUES?

When your main form of entertainment involves moving a joystick or gazing at a monitor, remember moderation.

While the theory that technology is bringing the world together may seem nice, research shows that the opposite is more likely to be true. In many ways, technology is actually drawing people away from one another, leaving them isolated and more prone to becoming depressed.

For example, researchers at Case Western Reserve University who studied the television-viewing habits of 2,000 adolescents found that those who watched the most TV were also the most likely to experience depression and anxiety. Another study, at Carnegie Mellon University, showed that people who spent the most time on the Internet experienced a significant decline in the sizes of their social circles as well as increases in depression and loneliness.

"When real relationships are replaced by bonds to technology, depression becomes increasingly more and more likely," says Robert Kraut, Ph.D., author of the Internet study.

Be aware that filling your life with technological forms of entertainment is often at the expense of beneficial physical outlets and face-to-face relationships, says Dr. Kraut. Make sure you balance daily high-tech experiences with enduring pleasures like tossing a football, hosting a potluck dinner, or joining a discussion group at a cafe or bookstore.

—Robert Kraut, Ph.D., *is professor of social psychology and human-computer interaction at Carnegie Mellon University in Pittsburgh.*

Diet, Herbs, and Supplements

"The tide is turning. Thanks to nutritional and herbal remedies, we are finally beginning to win the war against depression."

—Richard Brown, M.D., *associate professor of clinical psychiatry at Columbia University College of Physicians and Surgeons in New York City*

SINGLE OUT A GOOD MULTI

You load up on lettuce, manage to squeeze in milk—heck, you've even tasted tofu. But even with a healthy diet, you may fall short on some vitamins and minerals that affect your mood.

Nearly all Americans fail to eat the Daily Value of at least one vitamin or mineral, and many people don't get enough of two or more," points out Elizabeth Somer, R.D. You require these nutrients to maintain strong bones, keep your heart healthy, and much more. Besides the impact on your physical well-being, well-rounded nutrition is imperative for your mental health as well.

The solution? Continue to eat nutritiously and take a multivitamin/mineral supplement as insurance. A study of 129 healthy adults at the University College of Swansea in Wales found that those who took a multiple supplement daily for a year reported an improvement in mood and mental health.

And you don't have to buy the most expensive multi on the shelf. Just look for a single pill that contains 100 percent of the Daily Values for most vitamins and minerals. (Don't expect 100 percent of calcium, however, because it's too much to stuff into a tablet.) Also, choose a brand marked "USP," which means that it's held to higher quality standards than other supplements.

—Elizabeth Somer, R.D., *is a nutritionist in Salem, Oregon, and author of* Food and Mood: The Complete Guide to Eating Well and Feeling Your Best.

MAKE IT LIGHT

Sprinkle mini-meals throughout your day, and you'll keep your mind, body, and spirit in high gear even if you're not up to elaborate dining.

When you're out of sorts, it may seem overwhelming to spend an hour fussing in the kitchen to prepare that well-rounded supper—especially considering that when you're depressed, your appetite may be as well.

No matter how uninterested in food you are, though, it's imperative that you don't skip meals. You may not make the connection, but missing meals creates feelings of anxiety and emptiness that can only exacerbate depression. (Throughout this chapter, you will learn how the interplay of many subtle nutrients is essential to avoiding or overcoming depression.)

Some experts recommend thinking ahead by preparing multiple portions of soups or casseroles and freezing them for "down" days. Margaret Jensvold, M.D., has a favorite strategy: keeping the refrigerator stocked with no-fuss, easy-to-grab food and nibbling 250- to 350-calorie portions every 3 to 4 hours. Just be sure to grab your first mini-meal within 3 hours of waking, since skipping breakfast can worsen the blues.

Reach for mini-meals that offer both complex carbohydrates, which give your brain a soothing serotonin supply, and protein, which supplies amino acids that keep your energy up. Add three to five servings of fresh fruits and vegetables to the day's mix, get eight 8-ounce glasses of water or noncaffeinated beverages, and you can stay nourished without too much effort. Try to emulate simple combinations like these.

Mini-meal #1: 1 cup of low-fat plain yogurt mixed with ½ cup of blueberries or raspberries and 2 tablespoons of chopped peanuts or slivered almonds (290 calories).

Mini-meal #2: 2 slices of whole wheat bread spread with 2 teaspoons of peanut butter; wash it down with 1 cup of calcium-fortified orange juice (347 calories).

Mini-meal #3: Half of a sandwich made with turkey, reduced-fat Cheddar cheese, and lettuce, tomato, and cucumber slices and spread with 1 tablespoon of fat-free mayonnaise; top it off with an apple and a glass of water (291 calories).

Mini-meal #4: 12 baby carrots dipped in ¼ cup of low-fat ranch dip, 4 rye crackers, and ½ cup of your favorite juice (312 calories).

Mini-meal #5: 3 ounces of grilled chicken breast, 1 cup of steamed broccoli, 1 slice of whole wheat bread, and a glass of mineral water (270 calories).

Mini-meal #6: 1 pear, 2 fig cookies, and 1 cup of fat-free milk (280 calories).

—Margaret Jensvold, M.D., *practices in the Center for Life Strategies in Rockville, Maryland.*

HONOR YOUR CARBO CRAVINGS

Snack recklessly, and you'll feel worse.
Make informed choices, and you can
nibble your way back to bliss.

When we're down, we dream of happier times, when there were presents, favorite relatives, and . . . lots of cake. In fact, after a bad day, we can often think of nothing but hiding out with the cookie jar.

After all, our parents and teachers used sweets to distract us from sadness or to reward us for good deeds. But we seek foods that raise our blood sugar for reasons beyond the psychological underpinnings of "comfort food." Carbohydrates actually increase levels of soothing serotonin, the very brain chemical that many antidepressant medications are designed to boost.

So can you actually honor your cravings and indulge in a carbohydrate snack to improve your mood? As long as you understand that the kind of carbohydrates your brain wants is not necessarily the kind that first crosses your mind.

Complex carbohydrates, such as pasta, cereal, and whole grain bread, are what marathon runners load up on before a race to give them stamina. They are also what you should choose to answer your sugar cravings, says Peter Manu, M.D. Too many simple carbohydrates, such as table sugar, candy bars, and cake, can create both a nutritional and an energy deficiency, he says.

Think of simple carbohydrates as crumpled newspapers in your body's furnace. They burn fast and furiously but all too soon amount to nothing more than useless ashes. Before you feel any better, you've missed that burst of mood-lifting serotonin and maybe even lost some B vitamins that are essential for converting food to energy. What's more, getting into the cycle of trying to eat more high-calorie sweets—to regain that exhilarating burn after you quickly crash—can put on the pounds.

"Simple sugars are low in vitamins and minerals and may require more nutrients than they contain for your body to digest and process them," points out Dr. Manu. (When you're depressed, you often lack key nutrients already.) Complex carbos, on the other hand, are like long, steady-burning, seasoned logs that you can trust for your sustenance.

To use this dynamic to your advantage, grab a complex-carbohydrate snack once or twice a day to pick up your mood and your get-up-and-go. To help you avoid weight gain, the following power snacks have under 200 calories.

- 8 graham-cracker squares
- 2 multigrain waffles with 1 tablespoon of pure maple syrup or natural fruit topping
- 1 cereal bar
- 3 cups of popcorn
- 3 fig cookies

—Peter Manu, M.D., *is director of medical services at Long Island Jewish Medical Center and associate professor of medicine and psychiatry at Albert Einstein College of Medicine in New York City.*

EXIT THE "ZONE"

High-protein weight-loss plans may help you slim down, but they could also narrow your margin of happiness.

Chances are, you know someone who has dropped a few pounds on a diet that's sky-high in protein and forbids or restricts carbohydrates, such as The Zone or Atkins. But those plans can be anathema for people who have or are prone to depression, warns Judith Wurtman, Ph.D.

Since protein-based weight-loss plans severely limit the amount of carbohydrates you consume, your body can't make as much of the mood-regulating chemical serotonin.

If you're catering to your waistline as well as your mental health, Dr. Wurtman suggests cutting calories, not carbohydrates. For instance, if you slash 500 calories a day out of your diet, you'll drop about a pound a week (start exercising, and you'll lose even more). Here are five examples.

- Munch on an English muffin instead of a cinnamon-raisin bagel (savings: 256 calories).
- Top your baked potato with salsa rather than sour cream (savings: 25 calories per tablespoon).
- Order shrimp cocktail instead of Buffalo wings as an appetizer (savings: 218 calories per five pieces).
- Opt for a veggie burger instead of a quarter-pound hamburger (savings: 200 calories).
- Switch from whole to fat-free milk (savings: 64 calories per cup).

—Judith Wurtman, Ph.D., *is director of the Triad Weight Management Center at McLean Hospital in Belmont, Massachusetts.*

SNAP, CRACKLE, POP GOES DEPRESSION

Most ready-to-eat cereals are powerhouses of folate, a B vitamin that may stymie sadness.

Every time the medical community puts folate to the test, it seems that we learn another way that it can help people overcome feeling mentally dull and melancholy.

When Jonathan Alpert, M.D., and his colleagues gave 213 severely depressed patients 20 milligrams of fluoxetine (Prozac) for 8 weeks, patients with low levels of folate were twice as likely not to respond to the medication as those with normal levels.

It's also suspected that the nutrient may help you cope better with stress, since it supports your adrenal glands. "Falling short on this all-star nutrient can cause depression or exacerbate an existing condition," concludes Dr. Alpert.

One of the easiest ways to increase the folate in your diet is with ready-to-eat or hot breakfast cereal. The high achievers are Smart Start and Special K Plus (both with 400 micrograms) and Cheerios (200 micrograms). Wash your breakfast down with 8 ounces of orange juice for an additional 45 micrograms.

Dr. Apert also recommends talking to your doctor about taking a daily folic acid supplement of 1,000 micrograms, especially if prescribed medication isn't helping you feel better.

—Jonathan Alpert, M.D., Ph.D., *is assistant professor of psychiatry at Harvard Medical School and associate director of the Depression Clinical Research Program at Massachusetts General Hospital in Boston.*

THINK ZINC

While zinc's alphabetic placement makes it dead last on most vitamin and mineral lists, it should be at the top of your list if you have depression.

Since zinc is essential to many processes related to brain function, consider it essential for your mental health.

Falling short of your 15-milligram requirement for this mineral may lead to depression. Older adults and people with eating disorders are particularly vulnerable to depression from zinc deficiency, explains Hyla Cass, M.D., and they should discuss special requirements with their doctors.

To be sure you have your zinc requirements covered, take a daily multivitamin (most contain at least 15 milligrams) and eat foods rich in zinc such as lobster (8 milligrams per 3½ ounces), pork roast or lean beef (5 milligrams per 3 ounces), wheat germ (3½ milligrams per ¼ cup), and tofu (2 milligrams per ½ cup).

—Hyla Cass, M.D., *is assistant clinical professor of psychiatry at the UCLA School of Medicine and author of many books on natural health, including* St. John's Wort: Nature's Blues Buster. *She also answers natural health questions on her Web site at www.cassmd.com.*

LOSE THE LATTE

Don't expect caffeine to buzz away the blues.

When University of Michigan researchers studied 83 psychiatric patients, they found that the 22 percent who consumed more than 750 milligrams of caffeine daily (that's about 4 cups of coffee) were significantly more anxious and depressed than those who took in smaller amounts of caffeine.

A likely reason is that caffeine triggers the release of insulin into your bloodstream, which reduces your blood sugar level. Low blood sugar may lead to low energy and, ultimately, a bad case of the blues. In addition, caffeine may prevent you from getting a good night's rest, which exacerbates depression.

"Up to 35 percent of people with mild to moderate depression will feel better on a diet free of caffeine and sugary foods," says Larry Christensen, Ph.D.

Remember that caffeinated products include chocolate, coffee, green and black teas, colas, some root beers, orange or lemon-lime sodas, and over-the-counter pain medications. Here are some satisfying substitutes.

- Start your morning with minty herbal tea instead of coffee or other teas.
- Order fresh-squeezed juice or a smoothie rather than coffee at the bagel shop.
- Add a teaspoon of almond extract to milk instead of flavoring it with chocolate.
- Pour yourself a glass of sparkling mineral water whenever you're in the mood for soda.

—Larry Christensen, Ph.D., *is chair of the department of psychology at the University of South Alabama in Mobile.*

MELT THE CHOCOLATE CRUTCH

Experts warn not to cater to your chocolate cravings. Fortunately, there is another richly satisfying option.

Even if you're not sensitive to caffeine and you're at a healthy weight, relying on chocolate to chase away the blues is a bad idea, says Joseph Pizzorno, N.D.

While chocolate is rich in the mood elevator phenylethylamine, Dr. Pizzorno points out that the kick is short-lived. Once your phenylethylamine level starts to plummet again (usually within an hour or two, depending on how much chocolate you've consumed), you'll sink back into depression and crave—you guessed it—more chocolate. "It's a highly addictive mood elevator," says Dr. Pizzorno.

So, if you're prone to depression, does it mean that a Hershey's Kiss can never cross your lips again? Not exactly; just save chocolate for occasional treats like birthdays and anniversaries rather than using it as a frequent temporary fix.

To fill the "chocolate void," introduce yourself and your family to carob, an alternative that tastes similar to cocoa. Health food stores are likely to stock carob-flavored ice cream, carob-covered nuts, and carob baked goods. To make your own, try this wonderfully healthy recipe that uses carob in one of its most tempting forms—candy chips.

Oatmeal-Carob Cookies

1½ cups old-fashioned oatmeal
½ cup whole wheat flour
⅓ cup sesame seeds

⅔ cup toasted wheat germ

1 teaspoon baking powder

½ teaspoon salt

¼ cup natural peanut butter

¼ cup canola oil

¾ cup packed light brown sugar

¼ cup water

1 egg

1 teaspoon vanilla extract

1 cup carob chips

Preheat the oven to 375°F. Coat a baking sheet with cooking spray.

In a large bowl, combine the oatmeal, flour, sesame seeds, wheat germ, baking powder, and salt. Set aside.

In another large bowl, with an electric mixer on medium speed, cream the peanut butter, oil, and brown sugar until smooth. Add the water, egg, and vanilla and beat until smooth. Add the oatmeal mixture and carob and stir just until well-combined.

Drop the dough by rounded tablespoonfuls on the prepared baking sheet. Bake for 12 to 13 minutes, or until the cookies are golden. Let them cool slightly on the baking sheet, then place on a wire rack to cool completely.

Makes 36

—Joseph Pizzorno, N.D., *is a naturopathic physician and founding president of Bastyr University, which trains natural health practitioners, in Kenmore, Washington.*

REEL IN OMEGA-3'S

Many foods are teeming with the fatty acids that may protect you from depression.

Omega-3 fatty acids, the type found in cold-water fish, walnuts, and flaxseed oil, may protect you from both depression and heart disease, says Harold Bloomfield, M.D. In fact, people who live in countries such as Japan and Taiwan, where fish is the keystone of the diet, are six times less prone to depression than those of us in Western countries. One explanation is that fatty acids help regulate your body's production of mood-boosting serotonin.

Eat fish—particularly sardines, mackerel, bluefish, trout, albacore tuna, anchovies, salmon, and bass—at least three times a week. To boost omega-3's in your diet, try these suggestions.

- Order tuna sandwiches more often than pizza.
- Substitute salmon burgers for beef.
- Make a salad dressing with ½ cup of olive oil, ½ cup of flaxseed oil, ⅓ cup of freshly squeezed lemon juice, and 1 heaping tablespoon of mustard.
- Hold the meatballs and add steamed scallops, shrimp, and clams to your pasta sauce.
- Mix ground walnuts into yogurt and dough for home-made baked goods.
- Drizzle nutty-tasting flaxseed oil into hearty soups and onto hot breakfast cereals.

—Harold Bloomfield, M.D., *is a psychiatrist in Del Mar, California, and author of many books, including* Making Peace with Your Past.

STAY STEADY WITH FISH OIL

The fatty oils in fish may provide breakthrough relief for mood swings.

Researchers from Harvard University and McLean Hospital divided 30 patients with bipolar disorder (once known as manic-depression) into two groups. All of the participants stayed on their usual medications, but half took seven fish-oil capsules twice a day (for a total of 10,000 milligrams of the active ingredient), while the other half took olive-oil placebos. After 4 months, the mood fluctuations that characterize bipolar disorder eased for nine participants in the fish-oil group, but for only three taking the olive oil.

"We think that omega-3 fatty acids may prevent the transmission of brain signals that trigger moderate or dramatic mood swings," explains Andrew Stoll, M.D., author of the study.

Although larger studies are needed (and some are already under way) to fully understand the connection between fish oil and mood, Dr. Stoll suggests that you talk to your doctor about taking 3,000 to 10,000 milligrams of fish-oil supplements daily. They are available at health food stores and many drugstores.

People who have bleeding disorders, uncontrolled high blood pressure, or allergies to fish should not take these supplements.

—Andrew Stoll, M.D., *is a psychiatrist at McLean Hospital in Belmont, Massachusetts.*

CRACK A BRAZIL NUT TO SMASH SADNESS

Just one Brazil nut contains a hefty dose of mood-mending selenium.

Researchers from the USDA studied the effect of selenium on mood in 30 healthy men. For 15 weeks, half the group ate a diet that contained 240 micrograms of the mineral daily, while the other half followed a diet that supplied just 28 micrograms. The men on the high-selenium plan reported being less depressed than when the study began, while the low-selenium group felt just the opposite, says James Penland, Ph.D., author of the study.

A similar study by researchers at the University College in Swansea, Wales, also showed that selenium uplifted mood in patients who were given daily supplements.

Instead of rushing out to buy selenium supplements (especially since taking more than 400 micrograms a day may be toxic), Dr. Penland suggests that you increase your intake from food. At the top of his list of selenium-rich foods are Brazil nuts.

When you buy them in the shell and crack them at home, you can get about 100 micrograms of selenium in just one nut—for a mere 30 calories (precracked nuts contain 15 to 20 micrograms apiece). If you eat two nuts a day and also include seafood, whole grains, and poultry in your diet, you'll meet the daily 240 micrograms of selenium used in Dr. Penland's study with no sweat.

—James Penland, Ph.D., *is a research psychologist at the USDA Grand Forks Human Nutrition Research Center in North Dakota.*

CHEER UP
WITH ASCORBIC ACID

If you don't fit fruit and colorful vegetables into your diet, you probably get a meager supply of vitamin C—and getting an "F" on your C requirements can lead to depression and irritability.

Remember scurvy, the disease that mysteriously preyed on sailors—until they started taking vitamin C–rich fruits on board? It's probably no coincidence that depression is the first clinical symptom of scurvy, points out Melvyn R. Werbach, M.D.

In one study at the University of Leeds in the United Kingdom, the average vitamin C levels of 885 psychiatric patients were about one-third lower than those of 110 mentally healthy people. Here are some super-fast ways to stock up on C every day.

- Dunk baked tortilla chips into ½ cup of salsa (84 milligrams).
- Drink an 8-ounce glass of orange juice or eat one kiwifruit (75 milligrams).
- Cut half of a red or yellow bell pepper into slices and use them in a salad or sandwich (70 milligrams).
- Warm up a cup of tomato soup (66 milligrams).
- Add 4 ounces of Mandarin orange slices and 6 halved and pitted cherries to your salad (50 milligrams).

—Melvyn R. Werbach, M.D., *is clinical assistant professor of psychiatry at the UCLA School of Medicine and coauthor of* Natural Healing for Depression.

HARVEST YOUR NATURAL PRESCRIPTION

Many salad foods are packed with natural antidepressants. Mix and match some of these green ingredients, and you'll have blues busters in a bowl.

While almost all plant foods contain vitamins, minerals, and amino acids that may help ward off depression, some are more powerful mood improvers than others, says James Duke, Ph.D. Some of the best choices can be home-grown: Lettuce, pigweed, purslane, lamb's-quarters, watercress, rosemary, and thyme are all great. Lettuce, for instance, contains calcium, folate, lithium, magnesium, norepinephrine, phenylalanine, potassium, and tryptophan, all of which are compounds that fight depression.

And talk about a low-price prescription—greens like pigweed, purslane, and lamb's-quarters may be growing wild in your yard or local nature preserve. As long as the plants are growing where no chemicals are sprayed, and you are certain about their identification, you can let Mother Nature pick up the bill for your blues remedy.

Dr. Duke's suggestion is to toss these greens—or as many of them as you can find—into a salad. Top it with sunflower seeds, which are the richest food source of phenylalanine, an amino acid believed to combat depression. As for dressing, consider a citrus vinaigrette for extra vitamin C and great taste.

—James Duke, Ph.D., *is a former USDA ethnobotanist and author of many books on herbal healing, including* The Green Pharmacy.

DON'T OVERDO COCKTAILS

There are much better means than a
bottle of wine or a couple of martinis to
ease your troubles.

If you drink when you're blue, you risk the serious pitfall of self-medicating rather than getting the treatment that you may really need for depression. And considering what alcohol can do to your chemistry, drinking makes you feel progressively worse in the long run.

Not only is alcohol an antidepressant drug, but frequent drinking can also lower the level of omega-3 fatty acids in your nerve tissue, which aggravates depression. In addition, alcohol interferes with your body's regulation of the vital mood-boosting brain chemical serotonin, says Elizabeth Somer, R.D.

Her advice: If you're at a party and feel you that you can't be sociable without having a drink, ask for a wine spritzer. They generally have the least alcohol—and the fewest calories—of any alcoholic beverage. Of course, if you're taking antidepressant medication, alcohol is absolutely off-limits.

Whether you're hosting or attending a party, chances are you're not the only one abstaining. If it's your party, stock up on sparkling cider, sparkling grape juice, or an alternative punch so the "sober crowd"—including you—will have something festive to toast with. If you keep your mood steady by avoiding alcohol, you'll have all the more reason to celebrate.

—Elizabeth Somer, R.D., *is a nutritionist in Salem, Oregon, and author of* Food and Mood: The Complete Guide to Eating Well and Feeling Your Best.

HAVE AN HERBAL HAPPY HOUR

Instead of heading out to a bar after work (remember that alcohol only makes depression worse), have your friends over for nonalcoholic cocktails starring the relaxing herb kava.

Kava (also known as kava kava) is ideal for relieving anxiety-related depression, says herbal expert Kathleen Gould.

For decades, island cultures have used this herb to relax socially. Native to tropical forests, kava has long been a staple of Polynesian religious rites, where it is served as a fermented liquor. When it finally caught the attention of the medical community, clinical evidence began to stack up showing that kava can indeed balance your moods.

A review of seven studies by researchers in the United Kingdom found that kava significantly reduces anxiety levels. In fact, *every study* consistently showed a benefit—an outcome that's virtually unheard of in the research world, says Gould.

So what's the catch? "Well, kava can taste very bitter," Gould admits, "so I like to introduce people to it in a beverage that includes other tasty ingredients." Here is a recipe for one of her "kavatails." Drink up—and wind down.

Kava and Cream

    1 ounce kava kava root
    2 sticks cinnamon
    1 teaspoon cardamom seeds
    1 teaspoon grated fresh ginger
    1 teaspoon ground nutmeg
    2 vanilla beans, chopped
    1 gallon cold water
    1 quart eggnog or fat-free or low-fat soy milk
       Honey, to taste

In a large pot, combine the kava, cinnamon, cardamom, ginger, nutmeg, vanilla, and water (you can adapt the proportions to the number of guests you're serving). Cover and simmer for 30 to 60 minutes. Remove from the heat, stir in the eggnog or milk and honey. Strain the drink and chill in the refrigerator for 2 hours if you wish to serve it like a "'nog."

You can also purchase kava in capsules, and you can expect good results if you carefully follow the package directions. Never take more than is indicated, and never take it with alcohol or barbiturates. Also, since kava is a muscle relaxant, use caution when driving or operating equipment.

> **—Kathleen Gould** *is a professional member of the American Herbalists Guild and director of the Herb Corner and Learning Center in Melbourne, Florida.*

TAKE THIAMIN THERAPY

If you are a junk-food junkie, this B vitamin may be integral to lifting your depression.

Since most Americans get thiamin in a balanced diet, the tragic diseases and paralysis associated with severe thiamin deficiency are fortunately uncommon. But if you fall just slightly short, you may be troubled by fatigue, mental confusion, irritability, anxiety, personality changes, loss of appetite, and insomnia.

According to Derrick Lonsdale, M.D,. and to evidence from several medical studies, eating a lot of junk food can set your thiamin levels back enough to bring on these symptoms of depression. Foods that are refined or processed, for example, lose thiamin along with other nutrients when they are altered to make them lighter in color and texture, as is done with white flour. If you boil rather than steam foods, thiamin is released into the water, so it never has a chance to make it into your body. Moreover, drinking alcohol causes thiamin to be excreted with your urine, and the more sweets you consume, the more thiamin your body requires, since the vitamin is needed to help metabolize sugar.

Dr. Lonsdale suggests that you replace "empty calories" (refined sugars and processed foods) in your diet with fresh vegetables, whole grains (wheat germ, especially, is loaded with thiamin), and lean meats or legumes. If you aren't taking a multivitamin that contains at least 100 milligrams of thiamin, he also suggests taking a daily thiamin supplement.

—Derrick Lonsdale, M.D., *is a preventive medicine physician in West Lake, Ohio.*

HAMMER OUT OPTIMAL IRON INTAKE

Not getting enough iron in your diet may lead to anemia, a condition that can zap your zest for life.

If you follow health reports, you may be trying to do your heart a favor by cutting back on red meat. But when curbing meat or eating a vegetarian diet, you may need to beef up your iron intake to stave off depression, particularly if you're a premenopausal woman.

If you don't consume at least two or three servings of iron-rich foods daily, especially if you're a woman with heavy menstrual periods, you're at high risk for iron-deficiency anemia, warns Hyla Cass, M.D. One of the main symptoms of anemia is—you guessed it—depression.

In fact, more than 10 percent of 20- to 49-year-old women are deficient in iron, and about 5 percent have anemia, according to a study conducted by the Centers for Disease Control and Prevention in Atlanta. So to beat the blues and bolster energy, Dr. Cass recommends that premenopausal women talk to their doctors about taking iron supplements of 15 milligrams daily.

Men and postmenopausal women may not need supplements, but they also need to be savvy about getting sufficient iron. For example, consume nonmeat sources of iron daily if you eat a vegetarian-style diet, and pair those foods with foods high in vitamin C to maximize absorption, explains Dr. Cass. To get enough of this mighty mineral and be sure you absorb it, check out these terrific combos.

- Pair orange wedges with broccoli in a dinner salad (vitamin C: 111 milligrams; iron: 2 milligrams).
- Wash down a bowl of iron-fortified cereal with a cup of fruit or vegetable juice (vitamin C: 137 milligrams; iron: 4 milligrams, if you choose Cheerios and orange juice).
- Stir ½ cup of canned beans into a cup of tomato soup (vitamin C: 71 milligrams; iron: 3 milligrams).
- Toss your spinach salad in a citrus vinaigrette (vitamin C: 47 milligrams; iron: 3 milligrams).
- Have ½ cup of sliced strawberries with a bran muffin (vitamin C: 48 milligrams; iron: 3 milligrams).

—Hyla Cass, M.D., *is assistant clinical professor of psychiatry at the UCLA School of Medicine and author of many books on natural health, including* St. John's Wort: Nature's Blues Buster. *She also answers natural health questions on her Web site at www.cassmd.com.*

GET GOING WITH GINSENG

If the blues are turning you into a couch potato, you might need a charge from this herbal energizer.

I often recommend that patients with depression, especially people over age 45, take Korean or Chinese red ginseng (sometimes labeled Asian red ginseng) in addition to St. John's wort. It helps restore their energy," says herbal expert

Christopher Hobbs. For maximum effect, he recommends the following combination of herbal helpers.

Roots-and-Flowers Pickup Potion

½ teaspoon Asian red ginseng tincture
1 teaspoon St. John's wort tincture
1 teaspoon ginkgo tincture
1 teaspoon rosemary tincture
1 teaspoon lavender tincture
1 cup water

In a glass bottle, mix the ginseng, St. John's wort, ginkgo, rosemary, and lavender tinctures and the water. Drink ½ cup in the morning and the other ½ cup in the evening, but not within an hour of meals, for as long as you need a pick-me-up.

Alternatively, you may benefit from making yourself a cup of red ginseng tea daily by simmering 1 teaspoon of the ground root in 1 cup of water for about 20 minutes.

To avoid any dangerous drug interactions, do not use this formula if you are taking any prescription medications. You should not take red ginseng if you have high blood pressure; also note that it may cause irritability if taken with caffeine or other stimulants.

> **—Christopher Hobbs** *is a fourth-generation herbalist and licensed acupuncturist in Williams, Oregon, and author of* Herbal Remedies for Dummies.

KEEP YOUR EYE ON IODINE

Without this mineral, your thyroid won't function properly, and you'll be more apt to feel blue.

People who are deficient in iodine are very likely to suffer from thyroid-related depression, which is marked by fatigue and apathy, says C. Norman Shealy, M.D., Ph.D. Unfortunately, it's common for Americans to be iodine deficient.

It used to be easy to get plenty of iodine. You simply loaded your food with iodine-enriched salt, and you had plenty for days or even weeks. But since so many people are curbing salt intake to avoid bloating, high blood pressure, osteoporosis, and other health concerns, getting enough iodine is no longer as easy as a few shakes.

The best ways to get more iodine into your diet are to eat seafood at least three times a week and consider keeping a shaker of powdered kelp (available at health food stores) on your table instead of salt. It's not only an iodine boost, it also adds a nice flavor to soups, stews, and eggs and greatly complements most Asian fare.

—C. Norman Shealy, M.D., Ph.D., *is founder of the American Holistic Medical Association and director of the Shealy Wellness Center, an integrated medicine clinic in Springfield, Missouri. He has written several books, including* The Illustrated Encyclopedia of Healing Remedies.

GIVE A HIGH-FIVE TO B$_6$

*Like folic acid, this B vitamin plays an
important role in squashing depression.*

Approximately 60 percent of Americans fall short of the
Daily Value for vitamin B$_6$; among smokers, 80 percent
are deficient. Even a small deficiency can impact the production of serotonin, a mood-boosting brain chemical,
warns Karl Goodkin, M.D., Ph.D.

A review of studies in the *British Medical Journal* concluded that a B$_6$ supplement of 50 to 100 milligrams may improve depression associated with PMS. And many other
studies have demonstrated that B$_6$ supplements improve
mood in depressed patients.

Dr. Goodkin recommends that you start with a supplement of about 10 milligrams. If you don't notice an improvement after 2 weeks, increase the dose to 25 milligrams.
Still no effect? Raise the dose in 25-milligram increments
every few weeks until you reach 100 milligrams. Be careful,
however, not to exceed a total of 200 milligrams from a B$_6$
supplement and a multivitamin, because you may experience side effects such as a burning sensation in your hands
and feet.

In addition, it couldn't hurt to pump up the amount of
B$_6$ in your diet. Meet your daily requirement of 6 to 11 daily
servings of grains with winners like whole wheat bread,
brown rice, wheat germ, and barley. In addition, eat dark,
green leafy vegetables, chicken, fish, and nuts regularly.

—Karl Goodkin, M.D., Ph.D., *is professor of neurology
and psychiatry at the University of Miami School of Medicine.*

MEET SAM-E

Many depressed people are delighted to get acquainted with SAM-e (pronounced "sammy"), a supplement that may be able to stand up to prescription drugs.

SAM-e is short for S-adenosylmethionine, a compound found in every cell in your body. "I believe it works as well as prescription antidepressants, but it does it faster and with far fewer side effects," says Richard Brown, M.D. "Many of the people I have put on SAM-e have had dramatic responses. It's like you save their lives."

Unlike prescription antidepressants, SAM-e doesn't cause low libido and weight gain. What's more, many people who take SAM-e report that they feel much better within a week, compared to a month or longer with the prescription drugs. "SAM-e is a remarkable substance. It's one of the best weapons we have in the fight against depression," Dr. Brown says.

Plenty of scientific evidence supports Dr. Brown's personal experience. In a review of 17 studies conducted over a period of more than 20 years, SAM-e was found to be as effective as tricyclic antidepressants. And a study at the University of California, Irvine, compared SAM-e with the antidepressant desipramine HCL (Desipramine). More than 60 percent of the patients taking SAM-e experienced significant improvement, while only half of those on the prescription medication did.

Experts believe that SAM-e works to improve levels of serotonin, norepinephrine, and dopamine and to aid fatty acid function in nerves that are involved in mood regulation. If you're sure that you don't have bipolar disorder (formerly known as manic-depression), which SAM-e may actually worsen, Dr. Brown suggests that you talk to your physician about taking 400 to 1,600 milligrams of SAM-e daily (the dose used in most studies) for 6 to 12 months. If you're depression-free after that time, reevaluate with your doctor whether you need to keep taking the supplement.

To maximize its effectiveness, take SAM-e about 30 to 60 minutes before or 2 hours after a meal, and choose a high-quality brand. When Consumer Lab, a testing firm in White Plains, New York, evaluated the content of 13 SAM-e supplements, 6 were determined to be of poor quality. For a list of the best brands, log onto www.consumerlab.com.

Although only a few incidents have been reported, some people taking SAM-e have experienced indigestion and jitteriness. SAM-e may increase blood levels of homocysteine, a risk factor for cardiovascular disease. To reduce this risk, take supplements of vitamin B_6, B_{12}, and folic acid, which can lower homocysteine levels.

—Richard Brown, M.D., *is associate professor of clinical psychiatry at Columbia University College of Physicians and Surgeons in New York City and coauthor of* SAM-e: Stop Depression Now.

BUST THE BLUES WITH B$_{12}$

*While folic acid usually grabs all of the
B-vitamin glory in nutritional therapy
for depression, vitamin B$_{12}$ is an equally
powerful ally.*

Vitamin B$_{12}$ helps control your body's levels of homocysteine, an amino acid that you've probably heard about
in association with heart disease. So what does that have to
do with depression? Not getting enough B$_{12}$ cuts down on
the amount of homocysteine that your body can convert
into S-adenosylmethionine, an antidepressant compound,
explains Richard Brown, M.D.

You probably know S-adenosylmethionine better as
SAM-e, the mood-lifting supplement that is flying off store
shelves. But by loading up on B$_{12}$ and folic acid alone, you
may be able to naturally turn around depression and prevent a deficit of S-adenosylmethionine.

If dairy products and seafood are part of your daily diet,
you get a regular dose of B$_{12}$. But if you are a vegan (a vegetarian who forgoes dairy products), be certain that you drink
soy milk and eat meat-replacement products that are forti-
fied with B$_{12}$.

Dr. Brown suggests that you talk to your doctor about
taking 1,000 micrograms of B$_{12}$ daily—especially if you're
also taking a folic acid supplement, since folic acid can mask
a deficiency of B$_{12}$.

—Richard Brown, M.D., *is associate professor of clinical
psychiatry at Columbia University College of Physicians and
Surgeons in New York City and coauthor of* SAM-e: Stop
Depression Now.

SAMPLE MOOD-MENDING MAGNESIUM

Feel irritable and agitated most of the time? Perhaps you're not getting enough magnesium.

Magnesium is on the top of my list for fighting depression," says C. Norman Shealy, M.D., Ph.D. "That's because nearly everyone suffering from moderate to severe depression falls short of their requirements for this mineral.

"I've found that when I give people magnesium supplements, their depression improves. One of my studies showed that it helped 75 percent of depressed patients," adds Dr. Shealy.

He recommends taking a supplement of 375 to 500 milligrams daily. There are several forms of this mineral; look for magnesium taurate, which is easier to absorb than other forms. If you have heart or kidney disease, however, don't take magnesium without consulting with your doctor first. Also check with your doctor if you're taking other prescription drugs, especially to treat infections.

In addition to the supplement, Dr. Shealy suggests eating more magnesium-rich foods such as cooked spinach (155 milligrams a cup), almonds (105 milligrams per ¼ cup), cooked brown rice (85 milligrams a cup), cooked halibut (90 milligrams for 3 ounces), and kidney beans (70 milligrams a cup).

—C. Norman Shealy, M.D., Ph.D., *is founder of the American Holistic Medical Association and director of the Shealy Wellness Center, an integrated medicine clinic in Springfield, Missouri. He has written several books, including* The Illustrated Encyclopedia of Healing Remedies.

SEEK HELP FROM ST. JOHN

*These days, everybody from your boss to
your mechanic is talking about St. John's
wort to ease depression. But how much
of it is hype?*

Both conventional doctors and alternative medicine experts agree that *Hypericum perforatum*, better known as St. John's wort, is the premier herb to soothe depression. "St. John's wort is as effective at treating mild to moderate depression as prescription drugs. And it does it at about one-tenth of the cost and appears to do so without side effects such as low libido," says Harold Bloomfield, M.D.

Two reviews of studies support physicians' and patients' enthusiasm. Researchers from Ludwig-Maximilians University in Germany examined 23 studies from top-notch medical facilities. Of the 1,757 patients with mild to moderate depression studied, 50 to 80 percent of mildly depressed patients reported improvement in their symptoms and a general feeling of well-being while using the herb. And when researchers at the University of Hawaii conducted a similar examination, they concluded that St. John's wort performed as well as tricyclic antidepressants but with only half as many side effects.

The herb seems to work by enhancing serotonin and other brain chemicals as well as lowering levels of the stress hormone cortisol, explains Dr. Bloomfield. (When you're stressed, your adrenal glands secrete high levels of cortisol, which can dampen your mood.)

To minimize the chance of experiencing side effects,

such as nausea and increased sensitivity to the sun, Dr, Bloomfield suggests gradually increasing the dose over a few weeks' time to one 300-milligram dose three times daily. Many people prefer to take it with breakfast, lunch, and dinner, he says. As with prescription antidepressants, it can take up to 6 weeks to notice an improvement.

Check with your doctor before taking St. John's wort to be sure that any other supplement or prescription medication that you're taking won't interact. For example, if you are taking antidepressants, you shouldn't take the herb, because it works so similarly to fluoxetine (Prozac) and other selective serotonin-reuptake inhibitor (SSRI) drugs.

> **—Harold Bloomfield, M.D.,** is a psychiatrist in Del Mar, California, and author of many books, including Hypericum and Depression.

HEAL WITH THE HAPPY HERB

Latino cultures embrace damiana the way Europeans and Americans praise St. John's wort.

D amiana is considered the true happy herb, at least in Mexico, South America, and the southwestern United States," explains herbal expert Kathleen Gould. "It has such a good reputation that people seek me out to buy pounds of it at a time."

Damiana works to stave off mood swings by balancing your hormones. It also tones the central nervous system to ease frazzled nerves, says Gould.

She recommends one to three cups of damiana tea every day. Simply steep 1 teaspoon of the herb in a cup of hot water for 20 minutes, then enjoy the pleasant taste. For an extra herbal lift and taste, you may want to mix in a little lemon balm (which itself is called the gladdening herb). You can expect to feel better in a week or two.

> **—Kathleen Gould** *is a professional member of the American Herbalists Guild and director of the Herb Corner and Learning Center in Melbourne, Florida.*

ROOT OUT SLEEPLESSNESS

If you are plagued by insomnia due to depression or anxiety, try drifting off to dreamland by taking the herb valerian.

Valerian root exerts a mild sedative effect on the central nervous system. It not only helps you fall asleep quickly, it also provides deeper, more restful slumber, according to Janet Zand, O.M.D.

The herb has been widely studied in Germany since its sedative-inducing qualities, the valepotriates, were discovered in 1966. "Not only does the research support its effectiveness, but personally, I've seen it work on patients and even family members," says Dr. Zand.

If you've been counting sheep lately, she recommends purchasing capsules that contain 300 to 400 milligrams of concentrated valerian root extract, standardized to contain at least 0.5 percent of the essential oil. Never take more than the package indicates.

If you experience blurred vision, nervousness, headaches, irregular heartbeat, and nausea (all of which could be signs of a valerian overdose), stop using it immediately and consult your physician. Forgo this herbal remedy if you have any type of liver disorder or are currently taking any sleep-enhancing or mood-regulating medications.

—Janet Zand, O.M.D., *is a doctor of Oriental medicine and certified acupuncturist in Austin, Texas, and Santa Monica, California; cofounder and formulator of Zand Herbal Formulas; and author of* Smart Medicine for Healthier Living.

SMELL THE LAVENDER

Imported from Syria by ancient Greeks, lavender has been a popular home remedy for melancholy since the Middle Ages.

I tell my patients to use essential oil of lavender to raise their spirits, especially when they have stress, too," explains herbal expert Christopher Hobbs. "It's a quick pick-me-up." A study conducted by the Smell and Taste Research Center in Chicago suggests that the scent of lavender may lift depression because of its effect on brain waves. Lavender seems to trigger alpha and theta waves that are associated with relaxation and well-being.

Simply tuck a bottle of the essential oil in your purse or briefcase and take a whiff when needed. If you don't want to carry a whole bottle, dab a few drops on a handkerchief and sniff it whenever you need a lift. If you are like many people with depression and have an impaired sense of smell, you can sniff it many times a day to garner its effects.

Better yet, unwind in a lavender bath. Just fill your tub with warm water, add five drops of lavender oil, and swish it around. Soak until you're serene, but be careful not to slip when you get in and out of the bathtub.

—Christopher Hobbs *is a fourth-generation herbalist and licensed acupuncturist in Williams, Oregon, and author of* Herbal Remedies for Dummies.

INCREASE YOUR FLOW WITH GINKGO

You probably consider ginkgo biloba the memory herb, but it helps fight depression as well.

Poor circulation can dull more than quick thinking and sensation in your extremities. When people have insufficient circulation due to poor diet and other lifestyle factors, they are far more vulnerable to depression, says Janet Zand, O.M.D.

Combine the herb ginkgo with 45 minutes of aerobic exercise at least three times a week, and you'll be well on your way to increasing the flow of blood and oxygen to your brain. In a German study, people who received 240 milligrams of ginkgo daily showed significant improvements in mood, motivation, and memory within a month.

Dr. Zand suggests talking to your doctor about taking 80 milligrams of ginkgo three times daily. Be cautious about taking it, however, if you're taking anti-inflammatory medication, such as aspirin, or drugs that thin your blood, such as warfarin (Coumadin), because this herb may enhance this effect. Also skip the ginkgo if you're taking MAO inhibitor antidepressants such as phenelzine sulfate (Nardil) or tranylcypromine (Parnate).

—**Janet Zand, O.M.D.,** *is a doctor of Oriental medicine and certified acupuncturist in Austin, Texas, and Santa Monica, California; cofounder and formulator of Zand Herbal Formulas; and author of* Smart Medicine for Healthier Living.

REPLENISH BRAIN CHEMICALS

It doesn't have a catchy name like SAM-e, but 5-HTP may be the breakthrough supplement for you.

Research suggests that supplements of 5-hydroxytryptophan, or 5-HTP, offer impressive improvements for depression that's marked by anxiety, agitation, or aggression, says Melvyn R. Werbach, M.D.

This compound is derived from tryptophan, a feel-good amino acid found in protein-rich foods. It triggers the production of serotonin, the brain chemical that improves mood. Besides acting on serotonin, 5-HTP may also help trigger the release of other mood-boosting substances called catecholamines, Dr. Werbach says.

Talk to your physician about taking a 25-milligram supplement daily, he suggests. If you don't experience side effects such as nausea or nightmarish dreams, increase the dose over a month or two to 75 milligrams three times daily.

When choosing your supplement, be aware that some brands may contain a contaminant called peak X, which may cause serious symptoms associated with eosinophilic myalgia syndrome (EMS). The following brands don't contain peak X: Natrol, Nature's Way, TriMedica, Country Pride, and Solray. There have also been some reports of gastrointestinal distress, muscle pain, lethargy, and headaches.

—Melvyn R. Werbach, M.D., *is clinical assistant professor of psychiatry at the UCLA School of Medicine and coauthor of* Natural Healing for Depression.

Change
Your Mood
by Changing
Your Mind

"Happiness is something you can work at. It's a matter of identifying the things you do that get in the way of happiness and figuring out what positive activities you can do every day to augment it."

—David Lykken, Ph.D., *author of* Happiness: What Studies on Twins Show Us about Nature, Nurture, and the Happiness Set Point

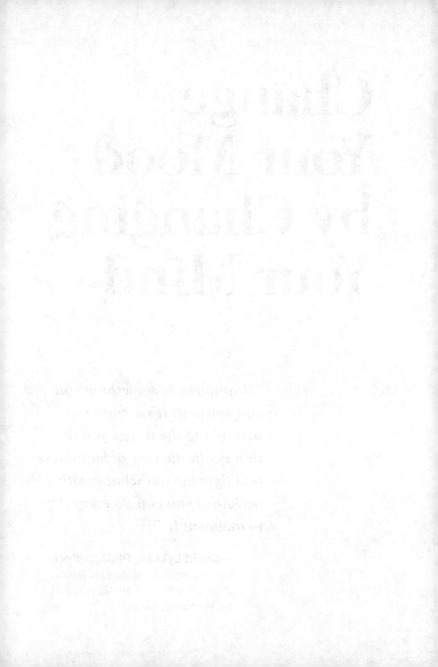

THINK OUTSIDE
OF THE BOTTLE

*Many of our problems can be solved when
we realize that our minds are creating
them—and that our minds can undo them.*

A popular phrase in business, encouraging people to solve
problems with a fresh approach, is "think outside
of the box." When it comes to resolving emotional turmoil,
Alice D. Domar, Ph.D., advises thinking outside of the
bottle.

Imagine that you have in front of you a large glass bottle
that contains a large, healthy, happy goose. How can you get
that goose out of the bottle without either breaking the
bottle or harming the goose?

Are you stuck? Here is a hint. You are approaching the
problem too concretely. Are you still stuck? Ask yourself
how the goose got in the bottle in the first place.

The answer to this question, which you may have spent
several minutes pondering, can be found in the initial posing
of the riddle, says Dr. Domar. Since the riddle only asked
you to *imagine* the goose in the bottle, all you need to do is
remove the goose in your imagination. Imagine the goose in;
imagine the goose out.

The point here is that many of our everyday worries are
as illusory as that goose in the bottle. We imagine in-
escapable traps that are nothing more than figments of our
worst fantasies.

The goose-in-a-bottle exercise is really a shorthand ver-
sion of cognitive restructuring. You can learn to stop in the
middle of a depressive episode and say to yourself, "Now

that's a goose in a bottle." Realize that the cause of your upset is purely a matter of perspective. Imagining that when you get home, you are going to have a fight with your husband, or that someone is not going to call as promised, are not problems unless you let them be.

> **—Alice D. Domar, Ph.D.,** *is director of the Mind/Body Center for Women's Health at the Mind/Body Medical Institute of Beth Israel Deaconess Medical Center and Harvard Medical School and author of* Self-Nuture: Learning to Care for Yourself as Effectively as You Care for Everyone Else.

DISPEL DISTORTIONS

To cognitive therapists, the cause of negative emotions is distorted thinking. Training yourself to think differently is your way out of the blues.

You need to recognize the traps that we all slip into in the form of distorted thinking. Once you learn to know the traps, bells and whistles should sound in your head to tell you to immediately back out of where your thoughts were going.

Cognitive therapy pioneer Mark Sisti, Ph.D., has identified some classic distorted thinking patterns for you to beware of.

All-or-nothing thinking. You see things in black or white. If you're not perfect, you think of yourself as a total failure. You make one mistake at work and decide that you are going to be fired. You get a B on a test and think it's the end of the world.

Labeling. This practice is an extension of all-or-nothing thinking. You make a mistake, but instead of thinking, "I made a mistake," you label yourself: "I'm a jerk." Your girlfriend breaks up with you, but instead of thinking, "she doesn't love me," you decide, "I'm unlovable."

Overgeneralization. The tip-offs are the words *always* and *never*. You goof up a punch line and say, "I always ruin jokes." You make a mistake and think, "I'll never get it right."

Mental filtering. In complicated situations that involve both positive and negative elements, you dwell on the negative. Your mother clearly enjoys the dinner party you threw in her honor but comments that the cake was a bit dry. You filter out all her positive comments and whip yourself for being such a lousy baker.

Discounting the positive. The tip-offs for this kind of distorted thinking are the phrases "that doesn't count," "that wasn't good enough," and "anyone could have done it." You do well on a test, and think, "It doesn't count; the test was easy." Your colleagues praise a presentation, and you think, "It still could have been better."

Jumping to conclusions. You assume the worst based on no evidence. Two of your coworkers are chatting at the coffee machine at work, but as you approach, they fall silent. Chances are, they simply finished their conversation, but you assume that they've been criticizing you behind your back.

Misfortune-telling. You predict the worst possible outcome. Your supervisor wants to meet, and you assume that you're going to be reprimanded. The sky is cloudy before a lawn party, so you decide that a thunderstorm is imminent.

Magnification. You exaggerate the importance of problems, shortcomings, and minor annoyances. Your toilet backs up, and you believe that you need to replace your entire plumbing system. A neighbor's dog tramples a few flowers, and you decide that your garden is ruined.

Emotional reasoning. You mistake your emotions for reality. "I feel nervous about flying, therefore, flying must be dangerous." "I feel guilty about forgetting my brother's birthday, therefore, I'm a bad person." "I feel lonely, therefore, I must not be good company."

"Should" and "shouldn't" statements. You play well in the company volleyball tournament but miss one shot, so you berate yourself: "I should have made that shot. I shouldn't have missed." You eat one doughnut and think, "I shouldn't have done that. I should lose 10 pounds." Other signals include *must, ought to,* and *have to.*

Personalizing the blame. You hold yourself personally responsible for things beyond your control. Your child misbehaves at school, and you think, "I am a bad mother." You are late for an appointment because of a traffic jam, and you think, "I am irresponsible."

—Mark Sisti, Ph.D., *is director of the Long Island Center for Cognitive Therapy in Suffolk, New York.*

ENCOURAGE THE PERSON IN THE MIRROR

If you let positive affirmations into your consciousness, they have the power to become more and more believable until, eventually, they may become real for you.

The practice of self-acceptance begins by learning to not judge yourself harshly and to believe in your potential. Your mind is an obedient servant that will help direct your life according to what you tell it, whether good or bad.

That's why metaphysical counselor Louise Hay encourages people to look into their own eyes and say something positive about themselves out loud every time they pass a mirror. Try saying, "I love and approve of myself now."

When you find negative thoughts resisting your positive affirmation, say to yourself, "Thanks for sharing, but now I have a new message for you," and repeat your positive affirmation, says Hay. Talk to yourself as you would your best friend.

You can also counteract self-defeating thoughts with affirmations like "I now release my need for depression," or "I now go beyond fears and limitations."

As many times as you can each day, repeat these words, or make up your own life-directing statements. The only rule is that you make statements in the present tense, such as "I am" or "I have," to bring them closer to reality.

> **—Louise Hay** *leads metaphysical study groups and empowerment workshops in Carlsbad, California, and has written many books, including* Empowering Women: Every Woman's Guide to Successful Living.

TALK YOURSELF OUT OF DISTRESS

Logic can calm you down and reveal solutions.

Take a close look at why you feel bad. Next, consider how to modify or "untwist" your thinking patterns so they don't lead you to misery. "The technique is quick and easy, and once people understand the basic concepts, it works for almost every situation," says Mark Sisti, Ph.D. Here is his method for approaching problems more constructively.

Step 1: Write things down. "Jotting down negative thoughts provides perspective and helps people detect distorted thinking more easily," Dr. Sisti says. If you are in a situation where you can't put pen to paper, he recommends doing the following steps aloud.

Step 2: Identify the upsetting event. What's really bothering you? Is it simply the fact that you have a flat tire? Or is it that you soiled your clothing while changing the tire? That you knew you needed a new tire but didn't replace it? Or that the flat made you late for your daughter's soccer game?

Step 3: Isolate your negative emotions. You may feel *annoyed* about the flat, *frustrated* that replacing it soiled your clothing, *angry* at yourself for not replacing the tire in time, and *guilty* for being late for the soccer game.

Step 4: Identify the negative thoughts that accompany your negative emotions. About failing to replace the tire, these might be "I always procrastinate. I never take care of things in time." About soiling your clothing: "I'm a slob. I can't go anywhere and look okay." About being late for the game: "My daughter will make a scene. She'll think I don't love her. And the other adults there will think I'm a bad parent."

Step 5: Identify the distortions and substitute rational responses. About the tire: "I don't always procrastinate. I juggle my job and family and accomplish just about everything that has to be done. I would have replaced that tire, but I had to deal with an emergency at work, and the tire just got by me." About the stained clothing: "I'm not a slob. I am usually very careful about my appearance, more so than most people, which is why things like this upset me." About the tardiness: "My daughter knows that I love her. She knows that if I'm late, whatever detained me was beyond my control. She's unlikely to make a scene, but if she does, adults will be there to comfort her. I've done the same for their kids and never thought of them as bad parents."

Step 6: Reconsider your upset. Are you still heading for an emotional tailspin? Probably not. But you still feel annoyed about getting the flat.

Step 7: Plan corrective action. For example, "As soon as the game is over, we're getting that tire fixed. That will take the time I planned to spend cooking dinner, so I'll pick up some take-out instead. It will be a nice break from cooking anyway."

—**Mark Sisti, Ph.D.,** *is director of the Long Island Center for Cognitive Therapy in Suffolk, New York.*

FORGE POSITIVE PATTERNS

We all think more than 60,000 thoughts a day, and the effective is cumulative. Be willing to change your words and thoughts and watch your life change.

What were you just thinking or saying? If you are nursing worry or anger or hurt or revenge, how do you think that idea will come back to you? In other words, if thoughts shape your life and experiences, would you want the ideas that are floating through your head today to become permanent truth? They do, more than you may realize, says metaphysical counselor Louise Hay.

Stop several times throughout the day and catch your thoughts. If you notice yourself saying something (to yourself or out loud) three times during the day, write it down. It has become a pattern for you. At the end of the week, look at the list you made, and you will see how your words fit your experiences.

This exercise will help you see that whatever we send out verbally or mentally has a huge effect on what comes back to us, Hay says. Life experiences may mirror our beliefs, but our beliefs also mirror our life experiences. Since the words you speak to yourself and others reinforce beliefs, it's largely up to you what fate you want to direct yourself toward.

If we profess that the world is a safe and joyous place, it's likely that we have encountered delightful friends and opportunities for ongoing growth. On the other hand, if we hold on to attitudes we were taught as children, such as "don't trust strangers," and "people cheat you," we may look and act so vulnerable that we have every reason to hide.

"If we want a joyous life, we must think joyous thoughts. After all, the key to controlling your life is to control your choice of words and thoughts," says Hay. Fortunately, even if you caught yourself professing negative patterns last week, that is in the past. What we choose to think and say today, at this moment, will create tomorrow.

> **—Louise Hay** *leads metaphysical study groups and empowerment workshops in Carlsbad, California, and has written many books, including* Empowering Women: Every Woman's Guide to Successful Living.

MAP YOUR ROUTE TO HAPPINESS

Learn to create and maintain a strategic plan that will liberate you from where you are stuck.

Sailors do not go out to sea without navigational charts and a sailing plan. We would certainly not drive across the country without a map. But most of us begin each day with little idea of what direction our hearts really want to go, much less how we plan to get there, says motivational leader Dannel I. Schwartz.

Start by writing down what can bring you the most joy and satisfaction. Figure out if it's a whim or if it is truly what you want more than anything else in life. Then, once it's settled, you can create a plan that shows you how to take a few steps each day to get closer to your dreams. Here are Schwartz's suggestions for getting started.

Monday. Think about how to do what you love and have it benefit others at the same time. For example, if you love to act, you might join a public theater company in your community—or better yet, form one.

Tuesday. Take your project idea and examine what is necessary in time, effort, and resources for it to become a reality. If you do it correctly, this project might become your livelihood, so take the time and effort to make the study complete.

Wednesday. Envision yourself doing this project. See yourself making mistakes as well as having fun and making good decisions. Imagine the details. For example, if you are an aspiring actor, see yourself reading a script at your first audition.

Thursday. Go to a library or bookstore or search the Internet to find three resources that will give you more information about the logistics of your project and will help you contact others who may be involved in similar efforts.

Friday. Make your initial "to-do" list. Plan the time that you'll need each day to work on it. Understand that all you have done so far is go through a planning process. In the weeks and months to come, you will have to do the hard work of making that project a reality.

Saturday. Tell someone you trust about your plan. Consider that person's opinions and ideas.

Sunday. To commit yourself entirely to the project, do something that will make it almost impossible to give it up, such as finally registering for a class or purchasing plane tickets.

—Dannel I. Schwartz *is a spiritual leader of Temple Shir Shalom in West Bloomfield, Michigan, and author of* Finding Joy: A Practical Spiritual Guide to Happiness.

"TIME TRAVEL" TO FORGIVENESS

Embrace who you once were and who you can become—to better appreciate who you are now.

You may have noticed that it seems easier to love and forgive others, especially children or younger people, for their shortcomings, than it is to love and forgive yourself. The following mind-shift meditation takes advantage of this insight, says Marcia Emery, Ph.D.

First, sit comfortably in a quiet place where you will not be disturbed, take several deep breaths, and allow yourself to completely relax. Recall an early memory from childhood, when you were in a state of innocence. Perhaps you were playing with friends or with a pet, grieving over a childhood loss or wound, or basking in the attention of a parent or revered elder. If that child were before you now, looking up to you in that state of innocence, how would you relate to him? You would probably embrace him with warm and tender affection, so do that now in your imagination—embrace the child that you once were with love.

Next, move forward to your early teens. See yourself in that time of biological change and emotional upheaval. See how you struggled to make sense of the world, feeling awkward and bewildered as the innocence of childhood seemed to vanish in the face of the complex social demands of adolescence. If the confused teenager that you were then stood before you now, you would probably feel compassion and want to help him through this difficult life passage. Express this compassion to your former self now.

If you are older than your midtwenties, move forward to

a time in your twenties when you were struggling to establish yourself as an adult, hoping to achieve some goal or fulfill a dream. Recall the ideals and the vision of life that inspired you. If that person were before you now, you would probably wish him every success and want his dreams to come true. Feel those feelings now for the person you were then.

Next, imagine yourself 10 or 20 years in the future. See yourself as older and wiser, having learned many life lessons and matured far beyond your present state. See that older, wiser you looking back on the person you are now. How would that person look at you? With at least as much, if not more, tenderness, compassion, and loving acceptance as you felt looking back on your past self. Do you think your future self would want you to judge and criticize yourself harshly now?

Embrace that wiser future self and digest, internalize, and absorb this mature, healing perspective. Any time you notice that you are judging yourself harshly, withholding from yourself the love that you deserve, give yourself a gentler perspective through time travel.

—**Marcia Emery, Ph.D.,** *is a psychologist in Berkeley, California; director of education for the Intuition Network; and author of* The Intuitive Healer: Accessing Your Inner Physician.

LET GO OF GRUDGES

It's never too late to release your offender and open yourself to healing.

Feelings of depression are often described as a pulling down or an uncomfortable heaviness. It's no coincidence that a denied need to forgive elicits the same sensations.

On the other hand, when you forgive, delightful physiological changes take place. You sigh and breathe more easily, your heart feels warm and light, and your blood pressure and heart rate drop.

Do you realize that it is possible to reap the benefits of forgiveness even when your offender is unreachable or even deceased? "You don't need anyone's permission to forgive," says psychologist Michele Wheat Dugan, "but it helps to trust in a loving presence to soften and open your heart." She offers this visualization for forgiving someone inwardly if external communication is either not possible or not preferred.

Allow yourself to relax fully for a few moments by breathing slowing and deeply. Then, as you exhale, begin by picturing your own heart, clouded—full of anger and bitterness. Imagine that it is a deep purplish color, which is the shadow energy of "lack of forgiveness." Then imagine an "ocean of forgiveness" that appears at the base of the heart and toward which the heart begins to tip gently, emptying out the bitterness and anger. Let your heart pour forth until all of its deep violet color is released into the sea.

The heart next becomes a luminescent violet and beholds another heart on the other shore (the person you want to forgive). Allow yourself to send forth your heart's light in the form of a rainbow to connect with that heart.

The heart on the other shore receives the light extended to it and also becomes brighter and more luminescent. In turn, it sends healing light back in the form of a rainbow. Together, the two hearts make a full circle of rainbow, half of which travels through the cleansing waters of the sea and half of which travels above the water, in the sunlight.

—Michele Wheat Dugan *is a licensed psychologist, workshop facilitator, and Dances of Universal Peace teacher in Kutztown, Pennsylvania.*

DECIDE YOU DESERVE

*If you believe that you are not worthy of
a happy life, you may keep yourself from
experiencing life's abundance.*

Sometimes, we refuse to put any effort into creating a
good life because we feel we don't deserve it, says
metaphysical counselor Louise Hay. The belief that we are
not deserving may come from our early childhood experiences. Perhaps we were told that we could not have what
we wanted if we did not eat all of the food on our plates,
clean our rooms, or put our toys away. Even as adults, we
may be compromised by unjust guilt based on someone
else's fears or bigotry. But you can learn to accept good,
whether or not you think you deserve it. Hay offers this
exercise to help you understand the power of deservability.

Answer the following questions as best you can, either
writing in a personal journal or speaking into a tape
recorder.

1. What do you want that you do not have? Be clear
and specific about it.

*2. What were the laws/rules about deserving that you
had when you were growing up?* Do you think your parents
and teachers felt deserving? What did they tell you? Did you
always have to earn in order to deserve? Did earning work
for you? Were things taken away from you when you did
something wrong?

*3. Do you feel that you deserve what makes you
happy?* Do you think, "Later, when I earn it" or "I have to
work for it first"? Are you good enough? Will you ever be
good enough? Or do you feel deep down that you deserve

nothing? Why? Where did the message come from? Are you willing to let it go? What are you willing to put in its place?

4. *Do you deserve to live?* Why? Why not? Did anyone ever tell you that you deserve to die? If so, was this part of your religious upbringing?

5. *What do you have to live for?* What is the purpose of your life? What meaning have you created?

6. *What do you deserve?* Continue to explore the roadblocks that came up in the later questions until you can repeat the following deservability statement and believe it: "I am not bound by any of the fears or prejudices of the current society I live in. The totality of possibilities lies before me. I deserve life, a good life. I deserve love, an abundance of love. I deserve good health. I deserve to live comfortably and to prosper. I deserve joy and happiness. I deserve the freedom to be all that I can be. I deserve more than that. I deserve all good. The universe is more than willing to manifest my new beliefs."

> **—Louise Hay** *leads metaphysical study groups and empowerment workshops in Carlsbad, California, and has written many books, including* Empowering Women: Every Woman's Guide to Successful Living.

CULTIVATE AN ATTITUDE OF GRATITUDE

This liberating mind shift will free you from negativity and increase all that is good in your life.

Gratitude is essential to the health of body, mind, and spirit. Remember, it is the nature of thought to increase. The more your thoughts are centered on what is missing, the more deficient you feel, and the more complaints you will utter. The more you practice gratitude, even in small ways, the more you are brightened by awareness of the abundance that life holds, an awareness that fosters emotional well-being and happiness. Wayne W. Dyer, Ph.D., offers some suggestions for cultivating the practice of gratitude.

Be aware of the need to be grateful for the suffering and struggles that are part of the fabric of your life. Sometimes, it's easy to simply be angry at your suffering, rather than to know it as a catalyst for your searching and awakening. Your ability to know the power of kindness and love most likely grew out of some pain and darkness in your past. Addictions teach purity. Anger teaches the ecstasy of love. Ingratitude teaches the need for gratitude. Hoarding teaches the pleasure of giving. Your own pain can teach you how to be more present and loving with others.

Begin and end each day with an expression of gratitude and thanksgiving. Each morning when you awake, you have been given the gift of a sunrise and 24 hours to live. This is a precious gift. You have the wonderful opportunity to take this day and live joyously, with appreciation for everything you encounter. Take a deep breath and be grateful for this exhilarating experience of breathing in life and love. Similarly, end your day with an expression of love, such as a repetition of the Hebrew word for peace, *shalom.*

Become a person who is willing to tell those around you how much you appreciate them. Make a concerted effort to say aloud how much you love your family members and friends, without making it a phony ritual. Be willing to say aloud what a lovely home you have and how much you appreciate it, or to express appreciation to someone who does a favor for you. Do this sincerely, and you will see how quickly the attitude is reciprocated and appreciated. The more you are willing to express gratitude, the more you cultivate an experience of unconditional love, which you know is the secret to manifesting all that you desire in life.

—**Wayne W. Dyer, Ph.D.,** *is a lecturer in the field of self-empowerment and author of many best-selling self-help classics, including* Manifest Your Destiny: The Nine Spiritual Principles of Getting Everything You Want.

Relax and Enjoy Life

"People who keep stiff upper lips find that it is damn hard to smile."

—**Judith Guest,** *American novelist*

FIND YOUR INNER KID

Children have gotten a happy-go-lucky nature down to a fine art. Let some of that joy rub off on you by spending time in their wonderful world of play.

Children play their way out of sadness, says John Morreall, Ph.D. As adults, many of us got out of the habit of playing years ago, but the kind of playfulness that comes so naturally to kids can zap mild depression.

"Most adults need a reason to play. They need an official vacation or a golf club in hand," Dr. Morreall says. Remind yourself that it's okay to laugh and be silly once in a while. Just an hour a week playing with a child, he says, can give you a different, more playful outlook.

If you don't have kids or grandkids, consider being a Big Brother or Big Sister to a child in need of a positive role model, or find a library program that needs volunteers to read to children. For information on volunteer opportunities, write to Volunteers of America, 1660 Duke Street, Alexandria, VA 22314-3421; call (800) 899-0089; or visit their Web site at www.voa.org.

Can't commit to volunteering? Grab a friend, visit a children's museum or a toy store, and try out the new gadgets. Maybe you can even show up the youngsters with your hula-hoop skills.

—John Morreall, Ph.D., *is professor of philosophy and religious studies at Old Dominion University in Norfolk, Virginia, and president of Humorworks, which conducts presentations and seminars on the benefits of humor in the workplace.*

HUMOR YOURSELF

Laughter is a natural lubricant that helps you release the intense grip you may have on misery.

When we joke about something, we restructure the situation in our heads. If you can laugh about your complaints, that's sometimes enough to snap you out of a mild depression, says John Morreall, Ph.D.

In fact, when the giddy aspect of life is put to serious medical study, research shows that humor is indeed good for our health. Along with physically reducing stress and even improving immunity, humor gives us an uplifting sense of control over our lives, says Dr. Morreall. Here are a couple of simple ways to tickle your funny bone.

• Make farce a habit. Routine can kill laughter, but breaking away from the mundane and doing something wildly different can be joyous. Leave your socks on in the bath, wear a funny wig to a friend's house, dress like your high school principal for a class reunion, or serve dessert first at dinner.

• Think like a comic. Woody Allen is a genius at hyperbolizing problems to the point of silliness. If you've had a particularly rough day, imagine how your favorite comedian would describe it to help take the sting away, Dr. Morreall suggests.

—John Morreall, Ph.D., *is professor of philosophy and religious studies at Old Dominion University in Norfolk, Virginia, and president of Humorworks, which conducts presentations and seminars on the benefits of humor in the workplace.*

HIT THAT JIVE, JACK

No matter whether your favorite tune is rock, rap, or romantic, music offers a potent way to be-bop the blues away.

Keep a sound grasp of the music that triggers happy memories, feelings, and thoughts, and you'll be well on your way to slipping into a better frame of mind, says Deforia Lane, Ph.D. In fact, right now, jot down a list of the 5, 10, or even 20 tunes that you find most uplifting. Then record them so you'll have a tape or CD that you can reach for at low moments in order to get yourself soaring again.

The key is to pinpoint the kind of music that strikes a happy chord in you. "Harp music may be very relaxing for some, but it reminds others of death," says Dr. Lane. She suggests music that reminds you of lighthearted times or childhood. A hint: The Vince Guaraldi Trio recorded the jazzy soundtracks for those lovable *Peanuts* specials.

—Deforia Lane, Ph.D., *is director of music therapy at the Ireland Cancer Center of University Hospitals in Cleveland.*

JOIN A CONGREGATION

When times are tough, let the healing embrace of a worship group lift you up.

People often turn to God in times of need, and research shows that group spirituality can actually keep depression at bay. In a study of 4,000 older people, researchers at

Duke University Medical Center in Durham, North Carolina, found that those who attended church frequently were about half as likely to be depressed as those who didn't.

Religious belief offers many people hope, says Michele E. Novotni, Ph.D. "It can be very healing and restorative because it takes you out of the immediate context of the here and now and puts you in the bigger fabric of life," she says. "You're no longer limited to that frustrating, this-is-all-there-is kind of mentality."

Beyond private prayer and spiritual reflection, though, the community itself is a wonderful healing body that can help people through tough times, says Dr. Novotni. Not only is the religious service usually very restorative, but you also have the opportunity to be around other people who are likely to be caring individuals. It can be very healing to do something productive to help someone else, says Dr. Novotni.

If you don't belong to a church or synagogue, take some time to visit different worship groups to find a place where you feel comfortable. Some people connect best to a formal service. Some prefer the charismatic, sing-and-dance-in-the-aisles approach. Others hear the spirit best in Quaker-style silence. "Remember, there are lots of different ways that people can connect with the Divine and express that connection," Dr. Novotni says. "You just have to find the one that feels right to you."

—Michele Novotni, Ph.D., *is associate professor of counseling at Eastern College in St. Davids, Pennsylvania; a licensed psychologist and certified school psychologist; and author of several books, including* Making Up with God.

REACH OUT AND TOUCH

Four hugs a day may keep the therapist away.

We all have the basic need to be touched. And when we're down and out, physical contact is an excellent natural prescription, says Judith Hall, Ph.D.

When nurses experimented with briefly touching certain patients but not others as part of their routine hospital activity, the female patients who were touched actually showed more favorable physiological and psychological improvements than the women who didn't receive contact.

Unfortunately, reaching out to others with a hug or a pat can be a touchy subject in this boundary-dominated society. If you're not sure what is appropriate for a particular relationship, it's usually best to defer to society's unwritten as well as written codes—like limiting quantity, for example. "One friendly touch or pat may be fine, but two in the space of an hour might not," says Dr. Hall. In general, "out in the open" hugs and strokes are more comfortable than those given, say, in a stairwell.

If you want the benefit of giving and receiving human contact but don't have the kind of relationships that offer it, consider joining a dance group, getting massages, taking Reiki (therapeutic touch) lessons, or volunteering as a "hugger" at the Special Olympics.

—Judith Hall, Ph.D., *is professor of psychology at Northeastern University in Boston who specializes in gender differences and nonverbal communication.*

VANQUISH YOUR VAMPIRES

When so-called friends start sucking the life force out of you, get out the psychological garlic and beat back those bad vibes.

Clinical psychologist Maryann Troiani calls them emotional vampires, and if you're feeling down, they're the last people you want to be around. "You can probably think of a few of these bloodsuckers right off the bat," says Troiani. "They're the people who put you down, criticize or mock you, or even sabotage your dreams. Friends who do nothing but complain or just fail to give you any support can also exact a heavy emotional toll."

If you think a relationship is worth the effort, tell the person specifically what behavior or attitude offends you. Explain that you will give him another chance, but that some things simply are not acceptable.

If your requests are disregarded, give yourself permission to burn some bridges. First, pull up the welcome mat by consistently turning down invitations from the bloodsuckers in your life. If they don't get the idea, you're going to have to come right out and tell them that you aren't interested in spending any more time with them.

If you can't completely discard these so-called friends, or if the vampire in question is a relative, Troiani's advice is to keep contact to a minimum. *Mentally* cut the cord, she suggests. "Remind yourself that their opinions don't matter anyway. They're just vampires."

—Maryann Troiani *is a clinical psychologist in Barrington, Illinois, and coauthor of* Spontaneous Optimism: Proven Strategies for Health, Prosperity, and Happiness.

ENLIST YOUR CHEERLEADERS

Ask your friends to remind you of all the things you have going for you when depression makes you forget.

When I'm low, I mention to friends that I feel like I am useless, and they reflect back to me some of my stellar accomplishments. It really helps to lift me out of that low feeling," says Marcia Emery, Ph.D. Even the smallest reminder can put a sparkle back in your eyes.

You can make a sort of game out of boosting your self-esteem with a group of friends, family, or coworkers. Give everyone a piece of paper and ask them to put their name at the top, then pass it to the person next to them. Each person should then write down one quality that he really likes, loves, appreciates, or admires about the person whose name is on that paper (but without adding his own name after the comments). Continue adding remarks and passing the papers until everyone ends up with their own.

It's sheer delight to see the way you touch others with your positive thoughts, as well as to be recognized for your own gifts. Keep the list somewhere special where you can see it every day.

If there's no group available, make your own list of what you like about yourself and what you are proud of achieving, from childhood to the present.

—Marcia Emery, Ph.D., *is a psychologist in Berkeley, California; director of education for the Intuition Network; and author of* The Intuitive Healer: Accessing Your Inner Physician.

PUT A LEASH ON THE BLUES

A four-footed friend can help you make remarkable healing progress.

A growing body of research confirms that having a pet may actually increase your quality of life as well as your life span. Researchers at the UCLA School of Public Health, for instance, found that patients who shared their lives with dogs required much less medical care for stress-related aches and pains than those who didn't.

"Stress is not so much overcoming feelings as denying them," says Joel Gavriele-Gold, Ph.D. If a pet can get you in better touch with your emotions, it will help you relieve some of that stress, he says.

Human contact helps fend off stress, too, and a pet can help you make the connection. While you are out walking Fido, it's only natural to meet and chat with others. Studies have shown that people tend to look at you in a friendlier way when you are with an animal. People in wheelchairs, for example, receive smiles rather than uncomfortable stares when they are accompanied by pets.

"When an animal comes over and licks you and wants to play, it's hard to stay totally self-absorbed," says Dr. Gavriele-Gold. Whether you own a German shepherd or a gecko, a parakeet or a Persian, as long as you bond, the therapeutic benefits are surprisingly similar.

—Joel Gavriele-Gold, Ph.D., *is a psychologist in New York City.*

FIND THE HOPE WITHIN YOU

Take a moment each day to treasure your spiritual self, and you'll bolster your resistance to the blues.

Meditation or prayer can help you cleanse anxiety, hopelessness, depression, and other negative emotions out of your body, says Patricia Norris, Ph.D.

To try a simple meditation, sit in a comfortable chair and take several deep breaths to help you relax, Dr. Norris says. When you feel serene, close your eyes and slowly repeat, "Let my heart be like the sun and shine without judgment on myself and everyone." If your mind starts to wander off to concerns such as whether you'll be able to pay your mortgage this month, bring your concentration back to the phrase. Do this meditation for 5 minutes at least twice a day or whenever you feel bitter, angry, or sad.

"The sun is a symbol. When you go outside, the sun doesn't ask, 'Are you good enough to receive my light today?' It just shines on everyone, no matter who you are or how you feel. That's how I think we should envision ourselves," Dr. Norris says.

—Patricia Norris, Ph.D., *is a psychophysiologic psychotherapist at the Life Sciences Institute of Mind/Body Health in Topeka, Kansas.*

MASTER MINDFULNESS

*Living "in the moment" is the most
immediate way to get more satisfaction
and peace in your life.*

Did you ever notice that when you're not rehashing the past, you're busy rehearsing the future? If you are depressed, your unruly mind has free rein to really brood. By bringing your focus to whatever you're doing, however, you can gain a greater sense of control over the present. You may find that even the most menial tasks you do as you go about your day can be relaxing and centering, says Roderick Borrie, Ph.D.

Mindfulness doesn't require having profound thoughts all the time. You simply have to keep your thoughts in sync with your body. That means that when you're folding laundry, put your whole self into making each fold perfectly even and take pride in the neat piles afterward. If you're doing the dishes, relish the sensation of warm suds on your hands. If you're mowing the lawn, think about the riot of vegetation around your house rather than about your stock portfolio.

Your mind is usually several steps ahead of your actions. It's often removed from what you're doing and busily seeking things to be depressed about. When you start to feel melancholy, you can shift your attention to the present rather than getting bogged down by "should haves" and "if onlys."

—Roderick Borrie, Ph.D., *is a psychologist at South Oaks Hospital in Amityville, New York.*

UNPLUG THAT TV

The fact is, you may be spending half of your free time getting depressed.

Have you ever really felt elated when you've turned off the TV after watching late into the night? asks Geoffrey C. Godbey, Ph.D. More likely, the lethargy and emptiness that you feel can be described as the opposite of what you feel when you're engaged in a creative, social, or spiritual experience.

According to the A. C. Nielsen Company, the average American watches 3 hours and 46 minutes of TV each day. That's bad news for the psyche, says Dr. Godbey. Research suggests that the longer you watch TV at any given time, the more your mood deteriorates.

One of the problems is that television is isolating. The average American household has at least two televisions, says Dr. Godbey, so watching has become a solitary activity that's not even broken up by conversation or comments about what's being seen.

The nonprofit organization TV-Free America suggests limiting viewing time to no more than a half-hour a day, or an hour every other evening. The group also advises moving the TV to a less prominent location in the house or covering the set when it's not in use. If you often have the TV on as background noise, use a radio instead.

—Geoffrey C. Godbey, Ph.D., *is professor of leisure studies in the department of health and human development at Pennsylvania State University in University Park and coauthor of* Time for Life: The Surprising Ways Americans Use Their Time.

TAKE POSITIVE STRIDES

*Pound the pavement often enough,
and you'll trample misery, stomp away
from anguish, and leave your blues in
the dust.*

An overwhelming amount of evidence links exercise and improved mental health, so you owe it to yourself to get off that sofa, lace up your walking shoes, and hit the road.

In one study conducted by David C. Nieman, Dr.P.H., a group of formerly sedentary women who walked 5 days a week for 45 minutes at a brisk pace reported improved moods within 6 weeks. Their enhanced mental outlook continued as long as they stuck faithfully to the walking routine.

For many, the social contact in group or partner workouts is an invaluable emotion enhancer. Experts continue to debate exactly why exercise keeps us happy, but they are quite sure that the newfound self-confidence that exercisers experience, the feel-good chemical endorphins that exercise activates, and the time out from a stressful routine that it affords all play a role.

Of course, it's not just walking that works. Studies have shown that other activities like cycling or swimming yield the same benefits. But for Dr. Nieman, walking is the sure winner. "I'm sold on it," he says. "It's so convenient. It can be done anywhere, any time. To me, there's no better exercise than walking."

—David C. Nieman, Dr.P.H., *is professor of health and exercise science at Appalachian State University in Boone, North Carolina, and author of several books, including* The Exercise-Health Connection.

GO WITH THE FLOW

*To rise out of a low mood, immerse
yourself in what makes you high.*

Psychologist Mihaly Csikszentmihalyi coined the term
flow to describe the kind of total absorption that a skier
might experience while racing down a snowy mountain or a
violinist might feel while tackling a challenging piece of
music.

The exhilaration of giving yourself so completely to an
activity frees you from the weight of your burdens, explains
Geoffrey C. Godbey, Ph.D. You can't expect flow to happen
with just any leisure-time activity, however (sorry, but sit-
ting in front of the tube won't do it). It usually happens with
activities that are complex enough to provide continuous
growth, says Dr. Godbey.

Moreover, whatever activity you choose to "flow" with,
immediate feedback is important. If you're painting, for example, the touch of your brush on the canvas makes a color
or an image appear. Your action should make something
happen that's reflected back to you.

Hobbies like gardening, crafting pottery, or working with
wood are all likely avenues for flow once you begin to master
them, says Dr. Godbey. You'll know when it happens. You'll
probably lose all track of time and won't care about making
a mess.

—Geoffrey C. Godbey, Ph.D., *is professor of leisure
studies in the department of health and human development
at Pennsylvania State University in University Park and
coauthor of* Time for Life: The Surprising Ways Americans Use
Their Time.

SEE THE LIGHT

It's not just plants that need light to thrive. So do we—and many of us just aren't getting enough of it.

Many people who have seasonal affective disorder (SAD) find that their symptoms improve with exposure to bright light. Extensive research shows, however, that they're not the only ones who could benefit from more light. Daniel F. Kripke, M.D., has carried out studies that suggest that light treatment has similar effects on all forms of depression, whether it's seasonally based or not.

Dr. Kripke's research indicates that increased depression among people who spend insufficient time outdoors is a universal problem. Even in a sun-drenched locale like San Diego, the average person spends less than an hour a day outdoors. Depression is less common in rural areas, says Dr. Kripke, and he believes that part of the reason is that rural people spend more time outdoors.

Not getting enough daylight isn't a problem only in winter, either. In Florida, light deprivation may be more likely during the hot, humid summer months.

If you have just a mild case of the blues, and it's convenient for you to spend more than an hour a day outdoors when the sun is high in the sky, that may be enough to brighten your mood. If the weather, fear of crime, or just workday responsibilities make that impractical, consider getting a light box.

When to use a light box is a subject of debate among scientists. Dr. Kripke believes that determining the optimal time has more to do with your waking habits than with whether the depression is seasonal or nonseasonal. If you wake early in the morning, he says, you may not need extra light until evening, so that's when you should use a light box. If you sleep late in the morning, you may need an extra light boost as soon as you wake, because you've already missed out on several hours of daylight.

The dose of light you need depends on how depressed you are. People with severe clinical depression may need 2 to 4 hours. For a mild case of the blues, a half-hour or an hour may be sufficient, says Dr. Kripke.

To use a light box, Dr. Kripke suggests putting it on your desk or next to your reading chair so you can get the benefits with very little disruption of your life. He defers to research findings that show that a light box is most effective if it's placed above your line of vision. Slant stands and lamps with tilt features are available to accommodate that position.

Use the light box for as long as you're depressed, advises Dr. Kripke. If you have chronic mild depression, you may want to simply incorporate it into your regular lifestyle.

—Daniel F. Kripke, M.D., *is professor of psychiatry at the University of California, San Diego, School of Medicine.*

GET GREEN TO LOSE THE BLUES

Nature in all its splendor can be a wonderful mood restorer.

Although much of the evidence of nature's restorative powers is anecdotal, it's certainly believable. We know that we feel refreshed when we take time to walk in the woods or bask on the beach. And countless poets, artists, and philosophers through the ages have documented the powerful effect of nature on our emotions.

Now, science confirms what our instincts tell us. In one study, 46 patients recovering from surgery in a Pennsylvania hospital were monitored to find out whether giving them rooms with views of natural settings would make them get better faster. It did. Those who had rooms with windows overlooking natural scenes stayed in the hospital for less time and took fewer painkillers than those in identical rooms with views of brick walls.

To make the most of our instinctive affinity for the natural environment, Roger Mannell, Ph.D., suggests getting out in it for an hour each day. It doesn't matter if you garden or birdwatch, kayak or play kickball in the park. And even if you're bound to home or office, you can "green up" your space with potted plants and even posters of outdoor scenes.

—Roger Mannell, Ph.D., *is a psychologist and professor of recreation and leisure studies at the University of Waterloo in Ontario and coauthor of* The Social Psychology of Leisure.

PICTURE A PERFECT DAY

Imagine if you could conjure up a happy ending to your woes. Well, you can. Use the following tactics and see how much better your days go.

Pretend that you know the world will end tomorrow. What would you do? Brood about what's missing in your life, or watch the sunrise, forgive grudges toward family and friends, and maybe take a personal day from work to run off to a baseball game or the beach?

Next, go a little further with the exercise. Write down what you'd do, then do it. "You'll probably do something constructive with your day, be more tolerant of others, and have a more hopeful outlook on life," says Redford Williams, M.D.

Now, what can you do to look forward to every day with this kind of excitement or contentment? Set aside a few minutes each morning to imagine the possibilities in store for you that day. If you are stuck in a dead-end job, for example, picture yourself interviewing for the job of your dreams. Or imagine yourself starting that running program.

Practice this imagery on your way to work. You can decide to either curse the traffic or give yourself something to look forward to.

—Redford Williams, M.D., *is director of the Behavioral Medicine Research Center at Duke University Medical Center in Durham, North Carolina, and author of* Anger Kills.

STAND TALL

Push back those shoulders and pull in that gut. Good posture not only looks good, it's an instant mental pick-me-up, too.

It's a fact: Unhappy, depressed people tend to slouch. Happy, optimistic people don't. "They take big steps, they walk faster, and they stand taller," says Maryann Troiani. "Pessimistic people shuffle their feet and take small steps." So walk taller, and soon you may feel your mood rise, too.

"There's a definite connection between the mind and the body here," says Troiani. "Just by changing your body posture, you'll instantly feel a little more optimistic, a little bit more confident, and more in control.

"Sometimes, when I felt overwhelmed, with too many things going on at the office, I would all of a sudden see myself slouching," she says. "Now, whenever I feel overwhelmed, I just straighten up a little bit and push my shoulders back."

If you really want to improve your posture, consider taking a class in martial arts, yoga, Pilates stretching, or the Feldenkrais method. The quality of your stance is, literally, the backbone of these practices. The exercises will also provide some depression-lifting social contact and give your body some physical stress release.

—Maryann Troiani *is a clinical psychologist in Barrington, Illinois, and coauthor of* Spontaneous Optimism: Proven Strategies for Health, Prosperity, and Happiness.

MAKE YOUR LIFE PEACHY

*Try adding the colors of the sunrise to
your life, and watch your mood get
rosier.*

Just think about it. When you're sad, you're "blue." If you're a Pollyanna type, you see things through "rose-colored glasses." There's no doubt about it, color and mood are inextricably linked. And if your spirits are in need of lifting, you should look to the warmer colors, says imagery expert Helen Graham.

As Graham explains it, the cycle of day and night affects us all. We tend to be more active in the early morning colors of red, orange, and yellow and progressively less active as the red tones slip out of the skies toward evening.

If you're feeling that your vibrancy needs a tune-up (particularly if you're prone to seasonal affective disorder) Graham's advice is to bring the colors of the sunrise into your life. Orange, in particular, is a very lively, energetic color. Since painting the whole living room orange isn't everyone's idea of good taste, though, you can use combinations of pinks and peaches. These colors are widely available and are highly effective when incorporated into home decor, says Graham.

> **—Helen Graham** *is a psychology lecturer at Keele University in England and author of several books on imagery and healing, including* Discover Color Therapy.

HAPPY VOICE, HAPPY HEART

Fake it with a cheerful voice, and your psyche may just fall for it.

A smiling face and a chipper voice may not always be reflections of inner happiness, but research shows that our psyches are willing to go along with whatever visage we present to the world. Even if you're feeling down, forcing a happy grin onto your face and a cheerful tone into your voice can actually turn your mood around, says Maryann Troiani.

In one German study, subjects who watched a cartoon while holding pens in their teeth (which caused their mouths to smile involuntarily) reported having much more humorous responses than did subjects who were physically prevented from smiling.

Troiani employs this phenomenon to jump-start a more positive outlook in her patients. "I remind people to look and sound cheerful, even if they feel bad," she says. "It's a simple technique, but there's a positive impact on the brain."

Not only will this convince your own psyche of its well-being, but when you speak cheerfully and appear amiable, people will react to you with more energy and charm than if you were gloomy. Then your mood can get the added boost of other people's joie de vivre. Misery may beget misery, but happiness is also reciprocal.

—Maryann Troiani *is a clinical psychologist in Barrington, Illinois, and coauthor of* Spontaneous Optimism: Proven Strategies for Health, Prosperity, and Happiness.

ARCH TOWARD BETTER DAYS

*You don't have to stand on your head
to reap the uplifting rewards of yoga.
Just do a little every day.*

Make a habit of practicing yoga daily, and you'll not only
get more limber, you'll also start to feel better about
yourself. Your blues may not vanish in an instant, but according to Carrie Demers, M.D., people tend to feel relaxed
and light after a yoga session. "Yoga integrates the mind and
body," says Dr. Demers, "and helps us be more comfortable
with ourselves."

The positions that are most helpful for lifting the spirits
are those that invigorate, stimulate, and energize, says Dr.
Demers. "Forward bends and poses where you fold in on
yourself aren't great for depression." What you want to look
for are the poses that arch your back and open up your
chest, such as the cobra, the camel, and the bow. "These
poses are deceptively simple," she says. "They look easy, but
if you hold them for several breaths, they will make your
heart pound and your body sweat."

For maximum mood boosting, do these postures every
day, says Dr. Demers. "It's more important to keep up with
yoga every day, say, for 15 minutes, than to do an hour-long
session each week."

The cobra. Lie face down with your forehead and the
tops of your toes touching the floor. Place your hands palm
down on the floor next to your armpits.

Next, look straight up as you inhale and lift your head
slowly off the floor. As you rise, let your spine curl to its

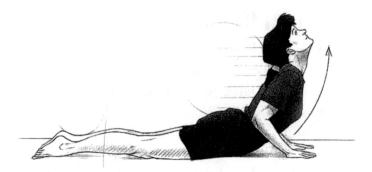

maximum degree, but keep your hipbones on the floor. Hold for several seconds.

When you are ready to slowly lower your body back to the starting position, let your stomach touch the ground first, followed by your chest and then your forehead, while you exhale. Repeat twice.

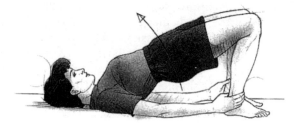

The camel. Lie on your back with your knees bent and your feet flat on the floor and hip-width apart. Grasp your ankles firmly, then raise and tilt your pelvis while you inhale. Breathe gently, holding the pose for several seconds.

To complete the exercise, curl your spine down, vertebra by vertebra, from top to bottom, and return to the starting position as you exhale. Repeat twice.

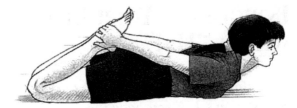

The bow. Begin by lying face down on the floor with your arms at your sides. Bring your feet up to your buttocks by bending your knees and grasping first one foot and then the other.

Lift your head and raise your thighs and torso as far off the floor as possible, pushing your hipbones down, as you inhale. Hold for 10 to 15 seconds while squeezing your buttocks and imagining your body as a curved bow.

To release the pose, let your chin touch the floor first, then let go of your feet and slowly resume the original position. Repeat this pose five times.

For more information on styles of yoga and locating an instructor, contact the Yoga Research and Education Center at P.O. Box 1386, Lower Lake, CA 95457, or log on to www.yrec.org.

—Carrie Demers, M.D., *is an internist and medical director of the Center for Health and Healing at the Himalayan International Institute of Yoga Science and Philosophy in Honesdale, Pennsylvania.*

INVIGORATE YOUR LIFE WITH A "HA!"

The "Ha!" breath can recharge and refresh you when you have the energy-sucking, low-down blues.

Ninety percent of your energy potentially comes from your breathing, says Marcia Emery, Ph.D., yet most people typically use only 10 percent of their breathing capacity.

Shallow breathing leaves you cranky, tired, and stressed out, but total breathing rejuvenates and regenerates. Engage life through your breath because breath *is* life.

Set your watch alarm to sound each hour, and make a "breath is life" check, says Dr. Emery. Are you relaxed and breathing deeply? Notice how any tense situation inhibits your breathing. Breathe deeply and participate more fully in life.

The following practice, the "Ha!" breath, is a dynamic way to recharge your body and mind with energy. It is like switching on your force field. Like the shout of a martial artist before delivering a strike, it generates a burst of chi, or life force, and is better than a lunchtime cocktail. You may want to do it at home or in your car on your lunch break, as it is apt to raise eyebrows, as well as the energy, in the office, says Dr. Emery.

To experience the "Ha!" breath, she says, sit or stand upright. Place your hands on your stomach just above your waist, with your fingertips meeting near your navel. Begin inhaling and inflating an imaginary balloon in your belly. Then exhale with an expulsion of air and shout, "Ha!" When first practicing this breath, you can push your stomach in with your fingertips as you exhale. Repeat the sequence five to seven times.

Next, close your eyes and observe how you feel in mind and body. Write down any observations. For example, you may feel a warm tingling in the center of your body, or you may experience an electric, energized state. This is common when deep stress is released from the pit of your stomach.

Many people feel like laughing while they are doing the "Ha!" breath. Some even break into spontaneous laughter—and as you know, laughter is the best medicine.

—Marcia Emery, Ph.D., *is a psychologist in Berkeley, California; director of education for the Intuition Network; and author of* The Intuitive Healer: Accessing Your Inner Physician.

FREE YOUR FEELINGS

Journal writing is a powerful way to write off pent-up anger, fear, and sorrow.

There's an uncanny alchemy about writing that is different from every other approach to catharsis and healing, including psychotherapy, talking to friends, and confessing to clergy, says Alice D. Domar, Ph.D.

Research at the University of Texas showed that people who wrote out their most painful thoughts and feelings for 20 minutes every day experienced marked improvements in their psychological and physical well-being. Unlike control subjects who wrote about trivial events, those who "hit a vein" reported that after just 4 days, they were less anxious and depressed, and they stayed healthier for as long as 5 months afterward.

Based on this groundbreaking research, Dr. Domar offers these tips for healing your wounds through writing.

• Sit at a table with a blank piece of paper in front of you (or use a keyboard) and, for 20 minutes, write nonstop about the most stressful event or ongoing problem that you face in your daily life. If you believe that your current problems are primarily the result of past events, write about traumatic circumstances in your past.

• You may choose to write about painful emotions associated with strained relationships, negative body image, sexual difficulties, money problems, spiritual distress, a frustrating medical condition, or whatever else is most pressing.

• Don't stop to correct your grammar or sentence structure.

• Write about what happened and how you feel or felt about it. The key is to not stick exclusively to either facts or feelings but to write about both. (Pure facts without feelings won't be liberating. Pure feelings with no facts won't help you understand your experiences.)

• Repeat this 20-minute process for at least 3 or 4 days, and make it a regular practice if you find that it continues to be fruitful. If you've covered one traumatic event or stressful circumstance, and you sense that there are others pressing, move on and explore them as well.

—Alice D. Domar, Ph.D., *is director of the Mind/Body Center for Women's Health at the Mind/Body Medical Institute of Beth Israel Deaconess Medical Center and Harvard Medical School and author of* Self-Nuture: Learning to Care for Yourself As Effectively as You Care for Everyone Else.

Alternative Options

When you're feeling low, it's comforting to know that there are gentle options like massage, uplifting herbal tea, and a spirited music therapy session to support you through the rocky times. Better yet, you'll find that alternative healers approach depression with the ultimate goal of resolving the underlying cause, so you can send symptoms away for good and improve your overall health in the process.

This chapter helps you determine which alternative modality is right for you and how to find more information on each option.

Acupuncture

We usually try to *avoid* getting a needle when we visit the doctor, but acupuncture is something else altogether.

For thousands of years, Asian medical practitioners have recognized and documented invisible channels in your body called meridians. But these channels can become blocked, preventing the free flow of life-supporting energy known as chi. According to Asian medical principles, when this happens, physical or emotional problems, such as depression, can result.

Acupuncture restores the flow of chi. As a bonus, it may also trigger the release of the natural mood-lifting chemicals serotonin, norepinephrine, and endorphins.

Acupuncture also helps you come to terms with your own emotions, according to John Myerson, Ph.D., a licensed acupuncturist and chairman of the Massachusetts Board of

Medicine Committee on Acupuncture. "With depression, you can close down and stop feeling, or you can turn anger and rage in on yourself," he says. "Acupuncture relaxes you, and when you're relaxed, you come out of your shell so you can feel positive again."

When you begin an acupuncture program, expect the practitioner to first take a detailed medical history. Then you'll lie comfortably on a table while the acupuncturist gently inserts thin needles—about the width of three hairs— just under your skin. Each session lasts from 25 to 40 minutes. A mild case of the blues generally requires two to four sessions, while more severe cases require more.

When looking for a well-trained practitioner, seek someone who's either licensed by your state or certified by the National Certification Commission for Acupuncture and Oriental Medicine (NCCAOM).

To find a qualified acupuncturist in your area, contact the American Association of Oriental Medicine at 433 Front Street, Catasauqua, PA 18032, or log on to www.aaom.org.

Craniosacral Therapy

If you're feeling blue, the answer might be to go with the flow—with craniosacral therapy.

Practitioners focus on the membranes that surround and protect the brain and spinal cord and the fluids that circulate within these membranes, known collectively as the craniosacral system. These fluids are in constant, tidelike motion, but sometimes this motion may be limited or immobilized—a situation that, according to practitioners, can affect your mental and emotional state.

"Experienced therapists are able to actually feel the craniosacral motion anywhere on the patient's body, in the same way that you can feel the heartbeat throughout the body," explains Kenneth Frey, a physical and craniosacral therapist and director of the Institute of Physical Therapy in New York City.

In people with depression, the restricted flow is usually near the base of the neck, the lower back, and the cranium. A practitioner will gently place his hands on these areas; this light pressure is said to restore the motion of the craniosacral fluids.

A craniosacral therapy session lasts 45 to 60 minutes, and the number of sessions required depends on the severity of the problem.

To find a qualified craniosacral therapist in your area, contact the Craniosacral Therapy Association of North America at 1214 Bellview Street, Burlington, Ontario L7S 1C7, Canada, or log on to www.craniosacraltherapy.org.

Eye Movement Desensitization and Reprocessing Therapy

Eye Movement Desensitization and Reprocessing, or EMDR, is a powerful new therapy technique developed to bring full recovery to victims of trauma, abuse, and other issues like insomnia and phobias that may be related to depression.

Using principles of REM sleep, the EMDR technique "unlocks" the negative memories and emotions stored in the nervous system and then helps the brain to successfully process the experience, says Carol Boulware, Ph.D., a clinical psychotherapist and an EMDR Level II Trained Therapist in Los Angeles.

The therapist works to gently guide the client to revisit the traumatic incident. When the memory is brought to mind, the client re-experiences the feelings in a way that makes it possible to gain the self-knowledge and perspective to resolve the emotional pain.

Typically, an EMDR session lasts from 60 to 90 minutes.

A history and evaluation are usually done in a few sessions. Then, in cases where a single, recent traumatic event is involved, a single session of EMDR may be all that is required. A more typical course of treatment encompasses between 5 and 15 sessions, usually on a weekly basis. After an EMDR session, there may be a strong sense of relief, a feeling of openness, or even euphoria.

To date, there are more than a half-million people worldwide who have benefited from EMDR therapy, Dr. Boulware reports. "EMDR is considered a breakthrough therapy because of its simplicity and ability to bring quick and lasting relief for most types of emotional distress."

Only practicing, licensed psychotherapists, psychiatrists, social workers, and counselors may receive EMDR training. Ask the therapist to provide you with his EMDR or EMDR International Association certification.

For information on EMDR therapists, contact Carol Boulware, Ph.D., 3130 Wilshire Boulevard, Suite 550, Los Angeles, CA 90401, or visit www.emdr.com.

Herbalism

It's true that an herbalist can prescribe herbs to directly elevate your mood, but if you consult an herbal practitioner, expect holistic treatment that goes beyond the obvious symptomatic relief, says Paul Bergner, clinical program director at the Rocky Mountain Center for Botanical Studies in Boulder, Colorado, and editor and publisher of the *Medical Herbalism Journal*.

For example, after a thorough review of your medical history and lifestyle, an herbalist may make the link that your mood is affected by liver function. If so, your remedy may include extracts of bitter plants that support the liver as well as changes in your diet. You may also receive a prescription for nerve tonics and gentle sedatives, such as extracts of oat seeds and kava kava to keep you calm while you sort out your problems.

There are no licensing or credentialing programs for herbalists in the United States, but the American Herbalists Guild (AHG) certifies practitioners who pass a peer review. They are then entitled to use the designation AHG as part of their credentials.

To find a qualified herbalist in your area, contact the American Herbalists Guild at 1931 Gaddis Road, Canton, GA 30115, or log on to www.healthy.net/herbalists.

Hypnosis

Put aside the notions of a cunning old guy swinging a pocket watch. In reality, hypnosis works with the will, not against it. "Hypnotists teach patients how to attain a state of receptivity in which the subconscious mind is open to helpful therapeutic suggestions," says Richard Harte, Ph.D., a cognitive-behavioral psychologist and hypnotherapist in New York City.

When you visit a hypnotist, he will ask many questions about your thoughts, feelings, and behavior, then will usually take you through three steps. The first is a letting-go process, where you get beyond the analytical, critical mind. As you sit comfortably in a chair, the hypnotist will instruct you to relax various muscle groups. As you start to focus on the hypnotist's voice, you may begin to feel different sensations, such as numbness, tingling, heaviness, or lightness.

When your conscious mind becomes subdued and your subconscious mind comes to the forefront, the hypnotist takes the second step—therapeutic suggestions. "I'll give suggestions to help the patient feel good about himself. Once he feels good, he can often handle problems on his own," says Dr. Harte. Finally, the hypnotist may teach you how to practice hypnosis on your own.

The entire process takes approximately four sessions. Look for a hypnotist with at least 100 hours of training, the amount required to be certified by the National Guild of Hypnotists.

To find a qualified hypnotist in your area, contact the National Guild of Hypnotists at P.O. Box 308, Merrimack, NH 03054-0308, or log on to www.ngh.net.

Intuitive Healing

If you want medication for depression or want to talk comprehensively about your problems with a psychiatrist, you first make an appointment with a physician. If you have a more esoteric sense that the life force behind your spiritual, emotional, or physical state is not glowing with the strength and radiance it could, you see a *meta*physician, otherwise known as an intuitive healer.

To an intuitive healer, maintaining health is based on having a strong primal life force, including the energy circulating around the body that holds the spirit inside, explains Malcolm Southwood, an intuitive healer in West Chester, Pennsylvania, and author of *The Healing Experience*.

Intuitive healing is an individual art, so no two healers work the same way. But in a typical 1-hour session, an intuitive healer will conduct a body scan by placing his hands slightly above your body to gain information regarding your distress (some healers evaluate you over the telephone). "If fear is involved, there's usually a feeling of heaviness around the stomach," explains Southwood. "It is as if there is a force that resists the hand moving through it."

Intuitive healers may attempt to free blockages or enhance low energy by sending you their own instinctive healing energy, which they identify as prana, chi, or simply, love. Others call on the aid of certain sounds, colors, and fragrances or their own massage techniques.

After a session, you may feel that something negative has been released, and, over time, observe that your coping skills have improved and your mood is better. You may also leave with assignments from your intuitive healer to practice specific self-nurturing techniques like affirmations or visualizations. You may leave with a clearer idea of how to bring more compassion and forgiveness into your life.

The United States has no national controlling body for training and licensing intuitive healers. Some practitioners have advanced degrees from metaphysically oriented schools; others learned as apprentices or attended classes with noted intuitive healers such as Caroline Myss, Ph.D. Southwood suggests using personal recommendations as your guide to finding a practitioner.

Your community may have a holistic health newsletter (ask at a health food store) where you are likely to find ads for intuitive healers. You can also locate an intuitive healer online through the World Organization of Energy Healers at www.healers.org.

Massage Therapy

You may think of it as relief for an aching back, but massage is also a great way to relieve emotional pain. It increases relaxation and decreases stress hormones such as cortisol, according to Denise Borrelli, Ph.D., vice president of the American Massage Therapy Association and owner of A Healing Touch Holistic Treatment Center in Medford, Massachusetts. It also improves overall physical health by flushing toxins from the system and improves overall psychological health by fulfilling our basic need to be touched.

Before beginning, a therapist should ask about any

health conditions that you may have, since people who have recently had head trauma or strokes should not be treated with massage. You'll then lie on a table (either clothed or unclothed and discreetly covered, as you prefer) and the therapist will administer his own style of rubbing, stroking, and pressing techniques. If the therapist is trained in safe touch, an approach that keeps the patient's safety and comfort in mind at all times, he will ask before working on a new spot so that you'll always know what to expect.

Sessions generally last an hour, and the number of sessions required depends on the severity of the blues. Massage therapists who have passed the national certification exam include the designation NCBMTB with their credentials. You may also want to look for members of the American Massage Therapy Association (AMTA).

To find a qualified massage therapist in your area, contact the AMTA Locator Service at (888) THE-AMTA (888-843-2682), or find them online at www.amtamassage.org.

Music Psychotherapy

Music's often-praised, soothing charms can help you beat depression. When you visit a music psychotherapist such as Diane Austin of Brooklyn, you'll be greeted by a wealth of musical instruments that anyone can play, from thumb harps to drums. You can choose the instrument that suits your mood and bang, strum, or sing out your feelings while Austin accompanies you on the piano or with her voice.

How does banging on a drum help you beat the blues? First, through music, you may be able to express emotions that you have trouble expressing through words. Second, when the therapist makes music with you or simply listens to you, you feel that your emotions are understood, sometimes for the first time. And third, because the music psychotherapist has training in counseling, he can help you understand the feelings that you express through the music.

If you aren't up to making a tune, the therapist may ask you to bring in a song that has special meaning to you so that you can listen to it and analyze it together.

Seek out a music psychotherapist who has a masters or doctoral degree in arts therapy or is certified by the American Music Therapy Association.

To find a qualified music psychotherapist in your area, contact the American Music Therapy Association at 8455 Colesville Road, Suite 1000, Silver Spring, MD 20910, or log on to www.musictherapy.org.

Naturopathic Medicine

A naturopathic doctor can offer a well-rounded program for resolving your depression based on advanced training in diverse alternative medicine therapies that include nutrition, lifestyle modification, natural medicine, and often hands-on treatments such as spinal manipulation and even acupuncture.

During your first visit, you may spend more than an hour telling the naturopath your medical history as well as details of the symptoms you've been experiencing. The doctor may also order lab tests to rule out any physical causes for your depression.

The naturopath will then create a unique wellness program to improve your overall health and happiness, explains Greg Garcia, N.D., a naturopathic physician and instructor at the National College of Naturopathic Medicine in Portland, Oregon. "Rather than focusing on individual symptoms like insomnia or anxiety, I believe greater success follows with treatment based on the whole picture of what the patient is experiencing," he says.

Your "prescription" for depression may include bodywork, amino acids such as tyrosine and phenylalanine, and homeopathic medicines. "Exercise is also one of the best treatments," says Dr. Garcia. "It's almost guaranteed to lift your mood."

He suggests choosing a practitioner who has attended a 4-year naturopathic medical school. Naturopathic physicians who are accepted into the American Association of Naturopathic Physicians (AANP) have attended medical school and studied the basic medical sciences in addition to courses such as homeopathy, spinal manipulation, and hydrotherapy.

To locate a naturopathic physician in your area, contact the AANP at 8201 Greensboro Drive, Suite 300, McLean, VA 22102, or at www.naturopathic.org.

For more information on these and other alternative healing modalities, contact the National Center for Complementary and Alternative Medicine at the National Institutes of Health (NIH). Write for their "General Information Package" at NCCAM Clearinghouse, P.O. Box 8218, Silver Spring, MD 20907, or log on to http://nccam.nih.gov.

Index